A WITCH'S GUIDE
To
SEXUALITY and GOOD
RELATIONSHIPS

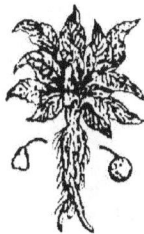

Tarona: To my husband for looking after the household whilst I worked with Howard on the *Witch's Guide* project

To Howard for time spent transforming my files and notes into *A WITCH'S GUIDE to SEXUALITY and GOOD RELATIONSHIPS*

Howard: To Jeanette

Acknowledgements

Grateful thanks to *Cherry Computers*, Faversham, Kent, for the excellent service and guidance. To Colin Barnard, *Polka Dot Art Centre*, Teynham, Kent, for his invaluable IT know-how and help.

SECRETS OF THE SEX WITCH

A unique perspective on human sexuality

Tarona Hawkins

With

Howard Rodway

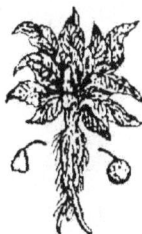

Mandrake

Published by

Mandrake

PO Box 250

OXFORD

OX1 1AP (UK)

Confidentiality Notice

Pseudonyms have replaced real names to preserve confidentiality and the privacy of those concerned.

Contents

Introduction

Secrets of the Sex Witch will be the most unusual sex handbook that you have ever read. This book is without a doubt unique. This is not an idle boast; it is a statement of fact.

Never before have the two subjects of sex and the occult been married in such an unusual way – and with sexual issues expressed as frankly as they are in this book. But let me start at the beginning.

Four years ago when I was discussing the subject of natural healing with practising witch Dr Tarona Hawkins, she mentioned during our conversation that she had notes, files and first draft chapters prepared about her psychic readings, counselling, past life regression work, magickal treatments and herbal remedies, all relating to clients' sexual problems.

Tarona Hawkins added that her reputation as a sex witch had gathered such momentum that most of her time was now occupied with sex counselling.

Tarona expressed the view that her knowledge, notes and records had immense value for those needing sex guidance, not only in the consultation room, but outside as well. She said she wanted her material transformed into a sex handbook and suggested we do it jointly. She asked me: "Would you like to look through my notes and records and see if you want to turn the material into a book?"

Intrigued, curious and sensing an unusual project, I could not resist responding to Tarona's suggestion. This volume is the end result of accepting Tarona's invitation to transform her records and her knowledge into *Secrets of the Sex Witch*.

Within this book you will find covered an incredible variety of sex and sex related subjects, for example:

Sex magick, sex massage, adult babies, fetishism, demonic sexual encounters, group sex, homosexuality, anal sex, sadomasochism, transvestism, transsexualism, sex feeders, sex for the elderly, impotence, penis enlargement, male hygiene, menstruation, past life traumas, the human sexual aura, sexual handwriting characteristics together with other sex related subjects.

To all those who read this book; individual members of the public, those with sexual problems, sex counsellors, and of course the occult community, it is hoped that through this book new insights will be gained into the unusually varied spectrum of human sexual behaviour.

In conclusion, let me state that in *Secrets of the Sex Witch*, pseudonyms have been used to preserve confidentiality and the privacy of those concerned. Even I do not know anyone's true identity because pseudonyms were in place when Tarona originally sent me the material for this book.

Howard Rodway

Section 1
The Old Religion and Sex Magick

1
Witches and Their Craft

Because this book is written from a witch's perspective, let me give you a pen sketch of what the world of witches and witchcraft is all about. This is for the benefit of those who are not familiar with the subject.

Witchcraft, also called Wicca, the Old Religion and the Old Path, is Britain's own native religion originating far back in time.

This oldest of spiritual paths has suffered extreme prejudice for a long time. In the main part fuelled by superstitious fear, this intolerance became rampant hatred during the medieval period when witches were burned and hanged in Britain and Europe. This prejudice has fluctuated but nevertheless remained constant right up until the present, and believe it or not, Britain's Witchcraft Act was only repealed in 1951.

Even today, a witch is often portrayed as a gnarled, bent and malevolent crone in a pointed hat, brewing unpleasant potions, perhaps with a toad or a black cat in attendance. This image is unfortunately still reinforced by Hollywood movies. The real world of witches and their craft however is as far removed from Hollywood as that town is distant from Stonehenge in England.

Witchcraft is a nature-based Goddess religion that holds sacred this planet, its animals, trees, plants and all life forms. Witches, like Native Americans, see themselves as guardians of Mother Earth and all her inhabitants.

Witches are the original environmentalists and animal rights supporters, and many witches encourage wild animals to live in their gardens as well as having cats and dogs in their homes. These animals though are not kept as sorceresses' apprentices. They are there because witches love animals.

Witches, who practise singly or in covens, are not just female. There are also male witches who, contrary to popular belief, are not called warlocks; they are witches, just like their female counterparts. The ideal balance in a coven is an equal number of males and females.

A coven is ruled by a High Priestess and her word is law within her group. A High Priestess, apart from being spiritually evolved, must have qualities of wisdom and leadership too for she is regarded as the earthly embodiment of the Goddess.

A witch will possess a number of skills that most often include reading the Tarot cards and Runes, compiling astrology charts, healing, casting spells and working with herbs.

A very important part of the witchcraft spiritual structure is a belief in the law of cause and effect, also known as karma. Witches believe that whatever someone does, whether it is a positive or negative thought or deed, that action attracts a reaction which is returned threefold to the individual concerned, either in this life or in that person's next incarnation.

As witchcraft is nature-based, it is also a fertility religion and its followers celebrate sex as a normal, joyful activity, without shame or prudery. Witches do not, let it be firmly stated, indulge in group sex orgies dedicated to Satan. First of all, witches do not believe in what to them is a Christian-created lord of evil, and secondly, witches' sex lives find expression outside the coven and in private.

Some excellent books have been written about witches and their craft including *Witch Amongst Us, Conversations with a Witch, Dancing with Witches* by Lois Bourne, *What Witches Do* by Janet and Stewart Farrar and *Drawing Down the Moon* by Margot Adler.

2

The Secret of Successful Spell-working

Within *A WITCH'S GUIDE* you will find some magick spells given for your use should you wish to use them. This space therefore is the appropriate place in which to dispel (no pun intended) the myth that a spell is just something quaint from your favourite fairy story.

A spell, whether it is chanted, written, acted out – or created with the use of herbs, oils or other material objects is, apart from the mystical aspect, an essential focus for your imagination as you visualize your desired situation being achieved.

No witch worth her bag of purification salt is going to waste time creating and performing supposedly pointless spells if they do not work, either for her, or for those who have sought her help.

Witchcraft to a large degree is about mind power and how that power can be utilized. If more people realized that they have within them the power to move mountains, they would indeed be creating their own reality.

Every true witch from an early age is aware of this power and how it can be used to change or create a desired situation. Your mind is your personal powerhouse, which, if used in a wise and positive way, will reward you and others in many amazing and miraculous ways.

But, sssh... This is all a secret, just between you and me. Remember that witches were burned and hanged for saying much, much less – and the burning times could return; after all, history repeats itself.

3

Sex Magick

Orgasm puts us into an altered state of consciousness and the special energy generated when we climax can be used for sex magick. The term sex magick therefore most often refers to the ritual leading up to the visualization of a desired situation at the moment of orgasm.

Witches have always known that in a spell-working context, sexual energy can be focused to bring forth a desired result.

Sex magick is best performed in your garden, in the countryside or on a deserted beach. A beach is one of the most powerful settings that you can choose. It must be emphasized however, that in any outdoor location, it is essential that you have total privacy. Sexual activity in areas used by the public is not, apart from the risk of breaking public decency laws, a good idea. A garden room, suitably furnished and fitted, can provide the ideal secluded space for sex magick.

To achieve good sex magick it is important to spend an evening with your partner. Go for a walk together through a wood or forest or even the darkened countryside. Hold hands and talk openly to each other about your wishes and dreams.

This is an ideal time to talk about your sexual fantasies. Discuss your joint desires and above all, make this period of time precious – and be attentive to your partner. Never talk about anything that is negative and never do anything that will make your partner unhappy.

If you are unable to go into the countryside or a garden room to perform

---

*See *Miscellaneous Information* for contact details of artists specializing in erotic art and sculpture.

sex magick, then use the bedroom of your home. Open your bedroom window wide and let nature's energy come to you.

Candles are an ideal addition to a magickal ritual. Light pink and red candles which should be placed in safe positions around the bedroom.

Your bed should be dressed in pink or red sheets to generate the energy of love and passion. You can also use pink or red pillows and cushions for the same purpose.

Mirrors often feature in sexual scenarios; let me warn you though, that you should not have a mirror at the bottom or the side of your bed. Mirrors in these positions are bad for relationships and often cause unfaithfulness. Overhead beams are not good for relationships either. If you have overhead beams in your home then I advise you to hang a crystal or wind chime from each one.

It is most important to remove from the bedroom any computer, television set or mobile telephone. These objects radiate electromagnetic waves that interfere with sexual energy. In fact, remove anything that distracts from the mood you wish to create. The exception can be a disc player playing suitably soft music. Your disc player, to be unobtrusive, can be hidden behind a potted plant such as a Boston fern.

What you really want in your bedroom are erotic paintings and prints on the walls, also ornaments or sculptures* of couples posed in sensual positions. Just remember that everything in the universe has an aura. It is important therefore that your bedroom expresses the appropriate vibration which is SEX.

Before you and your partner make love, have a shared or separate bath with some herbs and oil added to the bath water. My choice of oil would be either lavender or rose and my choice of herb would be rosemary. The ideal way to use the herb is to put a few sprigs in a cotton bag which can soak in the warm bath water.

After a bath, air dry your bodies naturally without using towels because towels collect negative influences from a floor or bathroom surface, then go with your lover to the bedroom.

Now try the sex magick feather massage in the next chapter.

4

The Sex Magick Feather Massage

Having made the initial preparations for your sex magick ritual as described in the previous chapter, now take it in turns to stimulate each other with the following feather massage, preferably using a red feather.

Beginning at the breasts, gently run the feather over the whole area of each breast, paying extra attention to the nipples. Then softly move up to the throat and across the shoulders and down each arm. Make slow and gentle movements and do not forget to include the inside of the elbows and fingers. Go between each finger and across the palm of the hand. Then gently trail the feather back up to the shoulders and down to the heart area. Now move the feather down to the feet, going between each toe and across the sole of each foot. Next, with an upward flowing movement, go from the sole of the foot back up to the heart and then to the head.

It is important that you pay attention to every curve and crevice of your partner's body – and the slower and gentler your touch, the more exciting it will be for your lover.

Explore every part of your partner's body, from the inside of the arms to behind the ears, not forgetting the back of the knees and between the toes. Treat every part of your lover's naked flesh as if he or she is a god or goddess.

The overriding thought that you should have at this time is the love that you each have for the other. Soon your sexual passion will begin to build up in your lower abdomen.

There does not have to be any particular sexual position in which to perform sex magick; however, it is better to position yourself so that you can gaze into your partner's eyes.

When you make love, make love slowly, becoming one person, then at the point of climax, concentrate on the joint venture that you both discussed earlier. For example, if you both want a green car, see the car in your mind's eye. See it parked in your driveway or outside your front door. Let your visualization cascade into the universe as you reach orgasm.

Do not worry if one of you should reach a climax before the other. This will not affect the potency of the magick.

And now some words of warning; only focus your energies on what you do want. Do not think about what you do not want or you will attract the latter.

When visualizing for gain, material or otherwise, remember the witches' ethic – that whatever you do, make sure your actions harm none.

Section 2
Private Sex Consultations

1
The Politician's Secret

During November 2003 I was at the famous *Erotica* show at Earls Court, London. This enormous three day event is always well attended for it is a festival that caters for every sexual preference – with the exhibition stalls selling everything from blue movies to fetish wear.

The 2003 *Erotica* festival was one of the most wonderful events that I had ever been involved with. The exhibition organizers really looked after their stall holders, even putting on a private party after the show ended.

There were many famous personalities at the festival and I gave psychic readings to a number of celebrities, including a well-known member of the British parliament.

This politician, who I shall refer to as Mr X, was middle-aged with a good head of grey hair. He was very charming and polite, and I immediately saw by the colour of his aura (the body's energy field) that he had been sexually abused during his childhood.

Mr X sat down in front of me and I held his hands and studied them. The first thing that I noticed was that he was sexually stimulated by pain and punishment. It was his little finger that revealed what would normally have been a hidden side to his sexual make-up. This finger was curved in a particular way, and whenever I see this characteristic, I know that I am dealing with someone who has an extraordinary fetish. Further on in this chapter I will go into more detail about this revealing feature.

After I had finished examining his hands, I selected my crystal ball to continue the reading.

The images that were coming at me from the crystal were amazing. I could hardly believe what I was seeing. This is what my crystal ball revealed about the politician sitting opposite me.

Mr X was walking out of the Houses of Parliament dressed in a business suit and carrying a briefcase. The image then changed to show the outside of another building. On the main windows of the premises was the wording *Special Sauna*. This was a brothel.

Mr X walked into the sauna's reception area where a large blonde woman was sitting behind a desk. They engaged in conversation and I saw money changing hands. The receptionist then got up from behind her desk and led the politician upstairs to a private room.

The next impression that came through was of a dark-haired woman in a flimsy dressing gown entering the room. She sat down alone on a bed. Mr X then came into view and stood by the woman. He was wearing a tight fitting black rubber dress and high heeled shoes. He was also carrying his briefcase.

The dark-haired woman spoke to him and Mr X reached inside his case and pulled out a rubber dress similar to the one he was wearing. He also took out a pair of bright yellow domestic rubber gloves. There was something different about these gloves though. It looked as if they had pins projecting from the fingers.

The next image was of the woman who had now put on the second rubber dress plus the bright yellow gloves. She was playing with Mr X's penis.

My crystal then cleared and gave me a vision of a headline in a national newspaper. The headline stated: **MP CAUGHT IN KINKY SEX**

SESSION. Looking Mr X directly in the eye, I told him about the newspaper headline.

Many years ago I learned to give a client every detail shown to me in a reading, even very personal details that the person concerned would not want revealed.

I had given the politician a full description of everything that I saw in the crystal. To my surprise he had not been at all outraged at what I had said. He had nodded his head and agreed, confirming that I had given him the correct information, adding that he often visited prostitutes at lunchtime.

I warned him to take extra special care or he would find himself exposed in the newspapers.

Mr X was a fetishist which is why he wore the rubber dress and rubber gloves. But the pins on the gloves also indicated that he was a masochist.

Fetishism is an attachment to an object with important sexual fascination for the fetishist. The object may not be directly sexual though. Often such fetish items are shoes, stockings or other items of clothing.

Masochism is sexual arousal gained through experiencing pain. Masochists can have various levels of desire, though some can only be aroused by experiencing extreme pain or torment. However, the masochist controls and terminates the session if the experience becomes undesirable.

The shape of a subject's hands will tell me a lot about his or her personality. In the case of Mr X he had spatulate fingers.

This distinctive characteristic told me that he was self-confident, energetic, and that he liked action. An unusually large Moon mount on his hand told me that he got sexually over excited and sometimes found it difficult to separate fact from fantasy. The politician's little finger curved away from his hand, an indication that he was not afraid of experimenting sexually and that he was likely to be deviant. Revealed too was that he was hiding what could probably be a big secret. I also saw that he might suffer in the future from mental illness. These characteristics were confirmed by the images that came to me from my crystal ball during Mr X's reading.

2

A Slave to His Feelings

It was over the airwaves that I first met Simon. He had phoned the radio station on which I was the regular psychic. Simon told me that he was a Virgo and asked me if I would give him a reading.

As soon as my caller started talking to me I had a clairvoyant picture of computers and fetish attire around him – and I could see the man shaking in terror. This was an unusual and interesting combination of psychic impressions but not suitable for discussion on a family radio show.

I gave Simon a quick general reading and asked him to contact me privately so that I could give him a more personal consultation. Simon accepted my invitation and phoned me in the evening.

Following on from the general reading I had given him during my afternoon radio phone-in, I told my caller that I had seen him looking very frightened. I asked him if he needed help or advice for any problems.

Without any preamble Simon told me that he had a deep rooted obsession about women being in control. He explained to me, "I want them to scare me and take away my freedom." He added that he wanted to be "humiliated and blackmailed" and needed a woman to control him. He admitted that he was ashamed of his desires and worried that his sexual obsession would reach the wrong ears, prejudicing his position at the computer company where he was the managing director.

Simon asked me, "Why do I need to completely give myself to a woman? Why do I want to serve her and be her slave and live to enjoy all the pain she inflicts upon me?" I asked Simon if he played out his slave role with a regular partner.

Simon told me that every so often he would spend a day in a massage parlour where, dressed as a slave, he would give his time freely to clean and dust the establishment until it was spotlessly clean. All he asked in return was to be told that he was owned and that his purpose was to serve his mistress. Part of this scenario was to receive painful punishment from his dominatrix.

Simon confided that his most exciting moment came when she took hold of his testicles and pulled him down on a bed. She would keep squeezing harder, at the same time ordering him to tell her that he was enjoying the pain, to which he would reply, "Yes mistress."

I asked Simon if he really enjoyed this pain. He told me that he did but that he was deeply troubled because he could not understand why he had a need to be humiliated in this way.

I explained to Simon that many people feel the desire at one time or another to be controlled or to control during sex, and that they become sexually aroused by the roles of submission and dominance which are the sexual companions of sadomasochism. I advised Simon that he should not worry about his activities so long as he was not accepting a harmful level of pain. I also advised him that for the sake of discretion he should confine his massage parlour activities to an establishment that was well away from his office and his professional colleagues.

There are many submissive males who are sexually stimulated by playing the slave role, either with a willing partner or a prostitute playing the dominant role.

There are a variety of ways in which submissive males dress for the part to act out their slave roles. Some like having clamps attached to their nipples and testicles – a painful pull on the clamps if the slave misbehaves – to dressing as a French maid, less knickers – so that a spank on a bare bottom can be administered when necessary.

In Luis Bunuel's classic French film *Belle de Jour* (1967) starring Catherine Deneuve, there is a marvellous humiliation sequence which goes wrong.

Deneuve's character is a sexually repressed housewife who, unknown to her husband, takes a day job as a prostitute in a Paris brothel. In the brothel she encounters one of the madam's regulars, a gynaecologist dressed in his slave role of a subservient butler who is about to be humiliated and punished for his clumsiness. This film sequence perfectly illustrates the submission-domination scenario. I will not give away any more of the story in case you see this excellent film.

The psychology of the sexually submissive personality, and please note that this will be a very broad one paragraph analysis of a complex subject, is that subservience allows the person concerned to let go of guilt. For example, anyone brought up in a very strict religious environment is likely to suffer from suppressed sexual feelings. Such feelings can find expression through a dominant partner who relieves the submissive from sexual responsibility.

3

The Home That Became a Haunted "House"

Commenting in the last chapter about the film *Belle de Jour* brought to mind the story of *Pillow Talk*, a haunted sex shop in Margate, Kent. This adult shop, according to some published accounts and confirmed by a *Pillow Talk* employee and ex employee, is haunted by the spirits of prostitutes who worked in a brothel that existed where *Pillow Talk* now stands.

These spirited females tend to appear when routine interior redecorating and maintenance work disrupt the shop's routine. The girls then cause their own disruption by trying on the shop's fetish wear and lingerie in the early hours - and leave the discarded apparel in disarray for the staff to find in the morning.

This story in turn reminded me of the time that I was contacted for a consultation by a "businesswoman" who wanted a reading, not for herself, but for her premises. She was worried that a spirit was active – and that was definitely bad for business. The business in question was the very personal service of a massage parlour in Leicester.

This tale first appeared as a brief ten line item in my book *Tarona's Ghostly Encounters* but the account created so much interest and curiosity that I am going to relate the full story here.

I made an appointment to check the massage parlour premises and when I arrived the madam was waiting expectantly for me. She took me through to her private lounge, sat me down in her comfortable lounge and made some coffee.

While I enjoyed a cappuccino she told me about her suspected ghostly presence before showing me over the house.

The building had rooms that oozed sex. The décor throughout was superb. Attention had been paid to every detail with murals of naked women emerging from the sea to create the right sexual vibration. She certainly knew about sex magick because erotically themed water murals and seascapes in bedrooms are wonderful for generating a mood of sexuality.

Hanging from the ceiling of one of the rooms was an amazing array of stockings and suspender belts. The bed was dressed in vivid red satin and the rest of the boudoir was furnished appropriately to give out the lustful energy of sex. Each room was very effectively themed, appropriately decorated and furnished, including the use of strategically placed mirrors and a skilled use of lighting.

The owner suspected that the haunted room was near stairs at the top of the building where a misty presence had been seen. It was the last area for me to inspect. This was a hideaway for "naughty schoolboys" and it was just big enough for a school desk and blackboard.

Once again the madam had hit the right note with the décor and furnishings, just perfect for those clients who wanted to be disciplined. The madam explained that she had been giving correction to a naughty boy in this room when they both felt an invisible hand touch them on the hair.

The owner was right in suspecting that this was the haunted area. There was an uneasy feeling about this particular room – and I knew that it had nothing to do with the sexual activities that took place there. The area was unnaturally cold too, an obvious indication of a ghostly presence.

The owner assured me that the central heating was switched on fully and I checked to see that it was. It was not really necessary to confirm because I had already picked up the presence of a spirit.

I told my client that her resident ghost was not malevolent but a prudish woman who I felt had used this room as her bedroom when she had been physically alive. She was making her presence felt because she disapproved of the use that her room was being put to. In her eyes her home had become an evil place. She was not at all happy.

The advice I gave to my client was to carry out a magickal cleansing ritual by placing an occult or religious symbol such as a pentagram or cross beneath the carpet. At the same time I suggested that she place plain quartz crystals throughout the house. And I also advised her to use another room for her "schoolroom".

The owner agreed to follow my advice and months later this massage parlour became one of the most successful in the area.

Going back to the tale of *Pillow Talk* in Margate, I am told that, surprisingly, there is no malevolent or broody atmosphere in the shop – just a rather peaceful and timeless mood about the place, rather like a library, so rest assured that if you visit *Pillow Talk* you have nothing to fear.

For those of you who may be worried about a spirit presence in your home or workplace, there are several ways of dealing with the situation.

Apart from the advice that I gave to the owner of the massage parlour, let me add some guidance that I always give to anyone who asks me for suggestions on how to deal with a haunting.

First of all, talk sympathetically to your resident spirit and acknowledge its presence. Making that kind of one-to-one contact is important because believe it or not, many spirits are more frightened of us than we are of them.

Secondly, when trying to help a lost soul return to the spiritual light, it makes sense to appeal to that soul's emotions, you can for example tell the entity that a loved one is waiting for them in the spirit world. Or, if you have no family background details about your ghostly presence, say gently - **You should no longer be here. Move toward the light**. You may of course be talking to a spirit who is perfectly happy to be close to the earth plane and thinks that you are the one who should move toward the light.

4

Two Virgin Swingers

On a Thursday morning in January, 2002, Jenny and Phillip arrived at my home for their erotic Tarot card reading. After we had introduced ourselves, I took the couple through to my psychic reading room.

On my table were the four packs of erotic Tarot cards that I would be using for the reading. Once we were seated comfortably around the table I asked Jenny and Phillip to choose one of the card packs. After a moment or two they chose a deck with a top card showing couples having group sex.

I asked them why they had been drawn to that particular pack. Phillip told me that he and Jenny enjoyed watching pornographic movies. They particularly liked films that portrayed group sex activities.

Both admitted to me that they found the thought of sex with others exciting but they did not want to ruin their marital relationship. Rather than cheat on each other, they felt that the answer was to join a swingers club. However, they wanted to have a reading to find out if swinging would put their relationship in jeopardy.

Before starting the Tarot reading, I asked them to visualize the following scene. The two of you are sitting together in a swinger's club. You Jenny will be wearing very brief underwear and stockings and you Phillip will be wearing a thong.

As you sit there, a strikingly beautiful woman appears who is adorned in a bikini brief. She walks over to Phillip, sits on his knee and starts to fondle him.

"How would you feel about that?" I asked Jenny.

"Cool, I think I could handle that okay", she replied.

Deliberately bringing the sensitive subject of penis size into my next visualization exercise, I said to Phillip, "Now imagine a very handsome man, with a penis twice the size of yours, who goes over to Jenny, puts his erect penis in her hand and asks Jenny if she would like to play with it. "How would that make you feel?" I queried.

Phillip's response was, "Just as long as we are both together when having sex with others it would be fine. Jenny often remarks, after seeing a well endowed porno actor that she would love to try a penis that size."

"Fine", I continued, "please tell me what you both think a swingers club will be like."

Phillip imagined a swingers club to be a very plush establishment with erotic pictures on the wall, and a friendly atmosphere with everyone talking to each other. But, above all, full of good looking young women with fantastic figures, all of whom would be looking for great sex.

I told Phillip that he was wrong. I went on to tell him that he could expect to find women in an age group from between eighteen to over seventy, varying in weight from seven to seventeen stone, and with breast sizes from quite flat to massive. Jenny's impression of a swingers club was that she would meet some stunningly good looking men with fit bodies.

I told Jenny that she too was wrong, that generally these clubs are full of middle-aged males. I added that some of these men have taken care of themselves and look great – but the average male swinger is not only fat but he has a beer belly too.

Continuing with the visualization, I asked them both to imagine being in a big play room in which they were on a huge plastic mattress with several other couples of all shapes and sizes.

Moving the focus of attention to Jenny I said, "While lying on the mattress, you Jenny suddenly have a woman sucking at one of your nipples. A moment later another woman starts to give you oral sex. How would that situation make you feel?"

Smiling, and not appearing to be alarmed by the thought of such a scenario, Jenny told me that she had "often fantasized about having sex with other women."

"Well, that's good to know because ninety percent of female swingers are bisexual", I replied.

Directing my next question at Phillip, I asked, "How would you manage with a sixteen stone woman?" Phillip pulled a face and told me that he was "not interested in big women and would not want to be in that predicament."

I then asked Phillip, "What if the fat woman's husband is handsome and Jenny liked him and they start to have sex. What would you do?"

Phillip shrugged his shoulders and replied, "I don't know."

So I addressed them both with the reminder that they had said that they wanted group sex. I added that they could not be selective when there were between ten to twelve sexually aroused naked couples on one mattress.

To soften the reality of group swinging, I told Jenny and Phillip to anticipate a time in the club lounge where they would probably meet a couple with whom there would be a mutual sexual attraction. This attraction would lead to the four of them going to a private play room and having a wonderful time.

I then asked Jenny and Phillip to cut the Tarot pack and select six cards each, and while doing so, to keep the cards face down.

Turning over Phillip's cards, I studied the images and predicted that he would have his first swinging encounter within a month. This would be with a woman born under the sign of Leo. I also saw that this confident and experienced woman would be good for Phillip.

Jenny's cards predicted that she too would have her first swinging session within four weeks. This would be with a Scorpio male who would please Jenny because of his stamina.

I could also see Jenny having her first bisexual encounter with a Libra female who will want to please her. I felt that it was going to be a memorable experience for Jenny.

Looking far into Jenny and Phillip's future, I could see them both becoming veteran swingers. They would stay together and have a long and happy marriage.

5

Secrets

of the

Sex Feeders

Have you ever wondered why some overweight people seem quite happy to be fat? That question is answered in this chapter as I invite you to enter the strange world of the sex feeders.

Some time ago I was giving a Tarot card reading to a woman named Jessie whose star sign was appropriately, Taurus. I guessed she weighed over 17 stone. She panted hard as she sat down in front of me, proof that she needed to lose a lot of weight.

I started Jessie's reading with the first card that I turned over which was *The Devil*. Whenever this card appears in one of my readings I know that the client concerned has a problem of a sexual nature.

As I concentrated on the reading I could see a large man giving Jessie a big box of chocolates and some cream cakes. I told her what I was seeing.

"Yes, that is correct, my husband buys these for me all the time", Jessie responded.

Moving a year or two into the future, I could see Jessie being told to lose weight because of a diabetic condition. I told her what was being revealed to me and gave her a warning to lose weight or face illness.

"That's impossible", Jessie said in response to my warning.

"Why is that?" I asked.

She replied, "Because my husband loves big women and he would go mad if I tried to lose weight."

I queried, "Even if it means your health suffering?"

She rolled her big dark eyes and commented that she and her husband loved food and she was not going to diet.

I responded by telling Jessie, "Fair enough, I am not here to judge you – but let me warn you that I see you housebound."

The rest of my client's reading concerned matters of a very general nature. Apart from the emphasis on food, there was little else that I could see in the cards for Jessie.

After I had finished the reading, Jessie told me that she and her husband were both sexually stimulated by food. She explained in detail that they both found body fat sexy. This woman openly admitted to me that her husband loved playing with her rolls of fat. She added that her husband liked being in control of her weight and her life.

Food is so sexually important to some couples that they will deliberately fatten themselves in order to enhance their sex lives. The more body fat they accumulate – the more they are sexually stimulated. The routine act of eating is also highly exciting to such couples.

Some sex feeders become so big that they become housebound and even bedridden. I could see Jessie in the latter situation and warned her that when she became bedridden she would find sex difficult, if not impossible.

Food is sexually stimulating to several different groups of people. The story of Jessie and her husband is just one example of a couple turned-on by food.

6

Two's Company.
Is Three a Crowd?

A good many of my clients have made appointments to see me for advice after seeing me featured on a television programme or after hearing me speak on the radio.

Such was the case with one who saw me on a Jo Guest television show. The programme was called *Sex Magic,* produced by Granada TV's *Men and Motors* satellite channel.

The day that filming was to take place was on a freezing Thursday in November 2002. The crew of four from *Men and Motors* arrived at my home before Jo Guest, so I took the group through to wait in the room where I had prepared some herbs and various other ingredients to be used in the show.

Jo arrived ten minutes later. She was a pretty, petite blonde with very large breasts and a big personality to match. She was naturally friendly and very down to earth so I took to her immediately.

The part that I was to feature in would show all aspects of sexual activity including bondage and fetishism. The mood of *Sex Magic* was to be somewhat tongue-in-cheek and light-hearted.

Programme presenter Jo Guest was a former British newspaper page three model and an adult movie star. Jo would travel the length and breadth of Britain to investigate a varied range of sex subjects. In fact, before coming to my home that day she had been filming a dominatrix (the dominant female in a sadomasochistic partnership), demonstrating the safe use of whips and other domination equipment.

The purpose of Jo Guest's filmed visit to see me was so that I could teach her to mix some potions and create a spell or two to attract a man into her life. The spells were simple and the ingredients were easy to obtain so that viewers could, if they wished, create the same spells without difficulty.

I felt that Jo would find love within months - and if my source of information was correct, Jo did just that.

The beauty of being part of a programme such as *Sex Magic* was that you could "lighten up" on some heavy sexual subjects, which had the effect, where I was concerned, of encouraging some troubled viewers to contact me with what to them would otherwise be strictly private problems.

And, it was not long after the programme was screened that I had a stream of phone calls, the first of which was from Martine, a woman who wanted to help her partner achieve his sexual fantasy which was to try a "threesome" – in other words, to introduce a third person to their sexual activities as an extra playmate.

Martine admitted that the thought of such a scenario turned her on. However, she was afraid that the reality would not match the fantasy.

I explained that a high proportion of men have such a fantasy, in fact a good eighty percent of males fantasize about three in a bed.

I advised her to thoroughly discuss the whole idea with her partner to ensure that he really wanted to realize his fantasy. I also mentioned to Martine that she must ask herself whether the threesome would also give *her* pleasure – and not just her partner.

My view is that if one partner is against introducing a third party, then the idea is best abandoned or, should the other partner be insistent, then just let that person go.

I have been contacted on numerous occasions by men and women concerning the subject of trios. Some of the men, believe it or not, have asked me if they should get their partners drunk before trying a threesome! My answer to that is a definite NO. Under no circumstances should anyone try to influence another by the use of alcohol or drugs. Nor should anyone ever use occultism to deliberately bind someone together in order to take away their free will. This is very dark magick and will incur heavy karma for the practitioner.

Apart from the problem of one partner for, and one partner against, a third party playmate, there are other aspects to consider too with this kind of ménage à trois situation.

If the suggestion from the male partner is to have another male make up the trio and he is adamant about this, then he may well be bisexual. It is better that this aspect of his possible sexuality is confronted by the female partner – sooner rather than later.

A suppressed bisexual man will often be turned on by watching a male have sex with his woman. This may be stating the obvious but it is often the obvious, which although staring us in the face, often escapes our attention – and our perception.

I have found that a man can be much more tolerant of his woman having fun with another female – than is the case with the reverse situation. A woman will often go mad if she finds that her man is bisexual. There are of course exceptions to the rule, and those of either sex who are really sexually liberated are often old souls.

Another sexual agenda for the male partner could be that he has lost some, or all, of his virility, so he becomes a voyeur and has sex by proxy - identifying and putting himself in the body of the other male as he watches the man have sex with his female partner.

If on the other hand he is happy to have both male and female partners at various times, his pleasure may well be from simple, uncomplicated voyeurism; the sexual excitement of watching others having sex.

An important point is to talk to your partner about exactly what you each seek from introducing a third party to your intimate activities. Couples must never forget that the person they invite into their home is another human being with his or her own agenda. Keeping this reality in mind goes a long way to avoiding hurt or unpleasant surprises at some future date.

With the above in mind, there are such feelings as jealousy and distrust to consider. One might think that such negative emotions would not enter a sexual arrangement that you have freely chosen but I am afraid this is not always the case.

As soon as you step over the boundary to experience group sex, nothing will ever be sexually and emotionally the same again. You cannot go back. You must therefore feel quite sure that each one of you is mature enough to deal with the emotional side of group sex.

So, let us assume that you have decided to go ahead and try a ménage a trois. You now want that third person. Perhaps you have a friend in mind or you move in circles where group sex is an accepted sexual lifestyle. All you then have to do is make the appropriate suggestion or offer an invitation.

If you do not mix with sexually liberated friends and acquaintances, you will have to spread your net a little wider.

You could for example advertise on the internet, in a contact magazine, or try a sex club which has singles nights. There are also swingers clubs which I mention in the chapter *Two Virgin Swingers*. But whatever route you take, please be careful. Caution is the key word and very necessary when dealing with this particular unknown x factor. It is really best if you can get a recommendation from someone who is familiar with the sex club and sex contact scene. One possible way could be to ask at your local (licensed) sex shop. The staff should be helpful if you are a customer.

If you and your partner already have an extra playmate, do be wise and keep the fact quiet from friends and family. I strongly emphasize this point about discretion because I have been contacted by couples who have lost their jobs – and been labelled as perverts by their supposed friends and treated as outcasts by their relations. I have also been contacted by those who have been secretly filmed at parties – who later found out that their filmed frolics were on sale from unscrupulous dealers who had used the internet as their market place.

My final advice for this chapter; have a sense of responsibility and never indulge in unprotected sex - and as I have said before, follow the witches' ethic, that whatever you do, let it harm none.

7

And Mother
Made Three

During the 1990s I was invited to give readings at a psychic party for a bride-to-be. What should have been an exciting and rewarding evening turned out to be an event that put me in an awkward and very delicate position.

One of those to whom I gave a reading was the mother of the bride. I had no preconceived ideas of what to expect from this person as she sat down in front of me.

I asked her to give me a piece of her jewellery and she gave me her wedding ring. As I held the ring, I soon saw flashing images of this woman with a dark-haired young man. I could see them parked in a field where they were having sex.

I told her exactly what I was seeing. She nodded in agreement.

I next saw the mother standing in the church with her daughter on the daughter's wedding day.

My next psychic impressions had me reeling and I wondered if I was getting false images. The man with whom she had been having sex was standing next to the bride. He was the bridegroom. This sequence was like a scene from the film *The Graduate* (1967) starring Dustin Hoffman and Anne Bancroft who played the sexually predatory Mrs Robinson.

I had no choice but to tell the mother what I was seeing.

She spoke softly and told me that for the past six months she had been having an affair with the young man. Neither her daughter nor her husband had any idea at all of what was going on.

I told her that I could see her daughter marrying this man and asked her if she did not think that the affair should stop.

"No," she replied, "I am in love with him."

When the reading came to an end she asked me not to tell her daughter what I had seen.

Because a reading is private, what had unfolded at the sitting had to be kept secret under the code of confidentiality. This therefore put me in an impossible situation, leaving me no choice but to give her daughter a false reading because I would have to omit what was going on behind her back. I hated myself for having to do this but to keep the peace I limited the daughter's reading to information about the wedding and general trivialities.

However, I did find the opportunity to ask her to look inward and ask herself if she really was in love with this man.

"Of course I am," she replied, "Why wouldn't I be?"

That evening I completed around five readings. I was so glad though when the party ended. I just wanted to get away from the deceitful situation that I had been confronted with.

Over the following weeks I put the family out of my mind – then several months later I got a phone call from the mother who asked me to give her a reading at her own home.

I agreed to give her a reading because I felt duty-bound to respond to her request. An important part of a psychic's code of ethics is to give advice regardless. Nevertheless, I went to the mother's home with reluctance and some misgiving.

Nothing had changed, for it was apparent that the mother's affair with her son-in-law was still going on – even after her daughter had married the man.

I told the mother that she was a fool and that no good could come of the affair but she was infatuated with her daughter's husband.

He was using her for what I believed was an obsessive fixation of having sex with his mother-in-law.

This was the first in a series of readings, following the initial party reading, that I gave the mother over a two year period. The rest of the readings were given at my own home and each sitting left me in a drained state after she had gone. There was a strange vibration about this woman and I always psychically cleansed my house after her visits.

Although I offered a number of spells to my client to help her terminate the affair with her son-in-law, she was just not interested. From her perspective, she was doing no wrong.

Two years after the mother's readings, and out of the blue, her daughter phoned me to book an appointment. How I was dreading seeing her.

When the daughter was with me having her reading, I calculated her number of influence and found that she was in a 6 cycle. This is a period that can bring either marriage or divorce. I saw from my Tarot cards that she had recently received a big shock. I could also see a divorce and a family breakdown. I told her what the cards were telling me. Surprisingly she did not look upset.

She responded to my comments by telling me that she had caught her mother *in flagrante delicto*. In plain English; the mother was caught red-handed having sex with her son-in-law. And in her daughter's bed too. As a result of this situation, the daughter had left her husband and her father had left her mother.

Although I understood that my client would be reluctant to trust another man, I assured her that all that had happened was for the best and that she would see this in retrospect. I also assured her that in time she would find genuine love, someone who really wanted her.

I plucked up the courage to ask my sitter something that had bothered me since the party reading. I said to her, "If I had told you about this affair that night, would you have gone ahead with the marriage?"

"Of course," she remarked seriously, "There would have been no way

I would have believed you." With that question answered I said farewell to my client after refusing to accept any money for the reading.

A few weeks later it came as no surprise when my intuition was confirmed with a phone call from the mother. She told me that the son-in-law had finished the affair, telling her that for him it had been nothing more than a sexual relationship. She wanted to know if he would come back to her.

"No," I told her as I put the phone down.

Obsessive relationships such as this, cause tremendous stress and unhappiness. There are many variations on the theme of obsessive emotional and sexual relationships, some so intense that they have ended in suicide and also motivated murder.

Here are some magickal spells to break an obsession.

To break an obsessive relationship

The walnut bath:

Put in your bath water six drops of *Walnut* from the *Bach Flower Remedies* range. As you get into the bath, visualize the person or persons you wish to banish from your life. As you visualize, repeat six times:

♦ Let this/these relationship(s) cease
♦ Let the connection(s) break
♦ A peaceful life for us I make

Now totally immerse yourself in the bath water and as you do so, see the subject of your spell being washed out of your life. After immersing and completing your visualization, stay in your bath for at least five minutes. Then step out of the bath and dry naturally without using a towel.

To keep a former lover from troubling you

Write your name on one half of a piece of red paper. On the reverse side of the paper on the other half, write the name of your former lover. Now fold the paper in two and tear it neatly through the middle. Save the piece of paper with your name on it but bury the half which has your lover's name inscribed.

For a peaceful separation from your lover

Take a small piece of rose quartz crystal and hold the stone up against the centre of your forehead where your third eye is located. Now visualize your unwanted lover moving away from you and going to a better relationship. As you visualize, say the following:

- ◆ Leave me now without delay
- ◆ And may the Goddess light your way
- ◆ As you tread a path away from mine
- ◆ Let new true love upon you shine

8

Sexual Encounters
of the Demonic Kind

The strange sexual encounters experienced by those featured in the following accounts were unlike anything that had ever happened to them before. Their unwanted sexual partners could literally be said to have come from another world – a world that witches refer to as the *lower astral*.

Over the years I have been asked to help with a variety of paranormal and ghostly happenings. Most of the ghostly activities that I have probed into have been straightforward – lost souls who have died tragically and not known they were physically dead. Such situations have been easy to deal with. Other spirit activity has fallen into a very different category indeed! Into that latter distinction fell four clients who initially contacted me by letter or via a telephone call, asking me for help with some very unusual personal problems.

Victoria

In the late nineties Victoria got in touch and begged for my help. She explained that she was being raped by an invisible force when in bed at night. And, during the day she often felt invisible hands groping her breasts.

Victoria told me that she always knew when "it" was around because of a pungent smell, like stale tobacco.

When I followed-up on Victoria's letter with a visit to her home, I could see that her unwelcome entity had attached itself to her aura.

I described what the ghost looked like and told her his name. Immediately the colour drained out of her face.

"That's my uncle," she said.

In eight out of ten cases where sexual intercourse takes place between a spirit and someone in the physical world, that victim has experienced sexual abuse of some description in childhood - or rape in adulthood.

Karen

Karen's first experience of sex with a demonic entity started with strange sounds and brightly coloured lights flashing before her. She told me her encounter was the first of many assaults that continued to take place – and spanned a twenty year period. This was really quite incredible.

When I went to see Karen she told me what the first assault was like:

"I could feel myself being pinned down to the bed and it felt like steel bands were wrapped around my wrists and legs. These bands stopped me from breaking free."

Karen explained that the sexual assaults she suffered were experienced both in the sleeping and waking state.

"There is always the sensation of a hand over my throat and I feel I am being strangled. I can then feel a muscular body pressing into me before he rapes me. Sometimes this sexual attack goes on for a very long time."

I asked Karen if at any point during her encounters she had enjoyed sex with her ghost. She told me that she had experienced multiple orgasms.

Karen admitted that she hated herself for enjoying the sex sessions with the entity but she had no control over her mind and body when the rapes occur.

Karen was a practising Christian who had prayed for help for years but no relief had been forthcoming – and her frightening astral attacker visited her at least once a week.

I told Karen that I was sure her fiendish visitor was an incubus – a Latin word meaning burden or weight.

According to many religious groups, incubi are fallen angels who have become demons. It is said that these - from good to bad spiritual shape-shifters fell from grace when they were angels because of their insatiable lust for women. As demons they continue to indulge their carnal appetite by raping and preying upon vulnerable women whose aroused sexual desires can only be satisfied by the incubi.

Ancient beliefs tell us that demons were spirits who came to Earth in two different ways. The first way for the entity to take shape and form was to occupy and activate a human corpse - and the second way was to appear as a recognisable person such as a husband, partner, friend or neighbour. If the female invited such an incubus into her bed, the entity had the power to put any other members of the household into a long, deep sleep.

The succubi are female demons who have sexual intercourse with sleeping men. Such a female, a succubus, features in my next account.

Ken

Ken told me that he was visited every night by a beautiful dark-haired woman. She had a Mediterranean appearance and possessed a perfect body with well rounded breasts and large nipples.

Ken's succubus would pin his hands to the bed and rub herself up and down his body until his penis became erect. The woman would then climb onto his erection and make love to him.

"It [is] the best sex I have ever known," Ken told me. "Making love to my wife seems dull in comparison and I have not much interest in sex with the wife these days," he confessed.

Due to Ken's lack of sexual interest in his wife, the cracks had started to show in his sixteen year old marriage.

Ken's wife was convinced that he was having an affair with a woman that he worked with, particularly after she awoke one night to see him moving his body in a sexual way. She was convinced that he was having sex in the dream state with his lover.

Mary

An elderly woman in her seventies called Mary asked me to help her.

She told me that she had a nightly visitation which would start with the bedclothes being pulled down. Then she felt a hand stroking her legs before it moved inside her thighs. Then the being, who she said was invisible, would have sex with her whilst she lay helpless on her back.

These four people, from different walks of life - and different age groups, had very similar sexual experiences - experiences that so disturbed them that they contacted me for help.

Many years ago I underwent training to be a nurse and social welfare carer. Part of my training was to be aware of any odd or dysfunctional behaviour exhibited by those in my care and to recognize such serious psychological conditions as paranoid schizophrenia. I also had to deal with individual cases of drug and alcohol addiction.

Over the years that past work experience has given me an invaluable extra tool with which to make personality assessments of those who see me privately.

In none of the four unusual cases mentioned in this chapter did I feel that the subjects concerned were suffering, or had suffered, from any clinical mental condition, nor did they exhibit any signs of drug or alcohol abuse. Without exception, they all functioned normally in a social environment and, apart from Mary who was retired, Victoria, Karen and Ken all had regular jobs.

I must of course make it quite clear that not all nocturnal, sleep state, bedroom sex experiences are to be blamed on demons! Sometimes, after dark nasties are nightmares indicating that the subconscious is reflecting some deep problem such as a hidden rape or some other traumatic incident from the past.

Doreen Valiente in her *An ABC of Witchcraft Past and Present* devotes several pages to the subject of incubi and succubi, including an interesting account of a married woman who was having sex with a spirit that spoke through her.

As an aside to the four demonic encounters that I have related in this chapter, the Hollywood actress Jayne Mansfield, who died in a horrific road accident in Mississippi in 1967, actually asked for a sexual encounter with an incubus according to Satanist Anton Szandor LaVey's authorized biographer Blanche Barton.

In *The Secret Life of a Satanist*, Blanche Barton recalls that Jayne Mansfield who was a priestess in Anton LaVey's *Church of Satan* as well as being personally involved with the Satanist, had been reading about incubi and, when down in Mexico to attend the Acapulco Film Festival in 1966, she phoned Anton to ask him to send her an incubus in his image to make love to her. He promised that he would, and Jayne then wanted to know how large the incubus' penis would be. She also wanted Anton to go into graphic detail about what the sexual encounter would be like.

Blanche Barton went on to tell her readers that on the following day Jayne phoned Anton to thank him for sending the incubus – followed by a specific description of what the sex had felt like.

Jayne Mansfield's association with Anton LaVey and the *Church of Satan* was dramatically terminated when her skull was crushed in the Mississippi car crash.

I shall end this chapter with a purification exercise for you to perform if you have unwanted visitors from the lower realm. This particular ritual is a good cleansing exercise generally – and particularly appropriate when you move into a new home:

Purification ritual

Fill up a small glass bottle (not plastic) with spring or filtered water. Add four pinches of sea salt to the water. Now cap the bottle and shake it so that the salt dissolves. Have the water standing by to use as the last sequence in the ritual.

Now light an incense stick (preferably frankincense) and have the burning incense ready in a holder.

The third and final item which will be the first to use is a white candle. Light your candle and put it in a holder.

Begin your house purification by stating out aloud, or silently, that through this ritual, all negative entities and energies will be banished and stopped from re-entering your home.

At this stage you can ask the Goddess for her blessing as you now take up your white candle and move to the front door, meditating upon the flame as you visualize it purifying your home.

Take the candle in a deosil (clockwise) direction, moving from room to room throughout the whole house – including the bathroom and toilet areas. Return to the front door with your candle when you have finished.

Now go through the same procedure with your incense stick. If your home has been host to negative energy or entities, see yourself in a much calmer state of mind as you sense the magickal ritual purifying every corner of your home. Return to the front door with your incense.

You finish the ritual exercise where you started – with your bottled salt water which combines the elements of earth and water.

Uncap the bottle and lightly sprinkle a few drops across the doorstep and on the door and then proceed in a deosil direction throughout the house, sprinkling a few drops of water in each room as you go, and at the same time, visualize yourself in a completely balanced state of mind. Return to the front door when the ritual is complete.

Remember to snuff out, not blow out, your candle at the end of the ritual, and take care at all times to ensure that the candle is not placed where it can catch something alight. Once your candle has served its purpose the remainder or stub should be thrown in flowing water or buried in the ground.

SECRETS OF THE SEXWITCH 48

You have now cleansed and balanced your home, and yourself, by calling upon the help of the four elements:

·**Earth** salt

·**Fire** candle

·**Air** incense

·**Water** Bottled salt water

With some of the magick spell rituals in this book, such as the one in this chapter, I often give guidance to move in a deosil direction. The reason for this is that in witchcraft moving clockwise is regarded as positive, whereas moving widdershins (anti clockwise) is regarded as negative.

There are exceptions to this rule but such exceptions do not apply to any ritual given in *A WITCH'S GUIDE*.

9

Anal Sex

In 1972 Bernardo Bertolucci's movie *Ultimo Tango a Parigi* was released amid a wave of controversy and moral condemnation, especially in his own country Italy, where he was indicted on charges of obscenity. Indicted with Bertolucci were the movie's stars Marlon Brando and Maria Schneider. Both actors were charged with participating in the making of an erotic film. So what was all the fuss about?

Well, anyone who has seen this movie, appropriately released in France as *Le Dernier Tango à Paris,* and in the English speaking world as *Last Tango in Paris,* will remember the simulated anal intercourse sequence in which butter was used as a lubricant.

What upset the Italian authorities, prompting them to indict Bertolucci together with Brando and Schneider, was not so much the eroticism, as such, in the movie, but the fact that prominence was given to anal sex, a birth control practice that has always been part of the sexual culture of people in countries officially discouraging just that – birth control. For that main reason *Last Tango in Paris* did not please the Vatican.

Last Tango made a controversial sexual subject very public, a subject that is still controversial and an area of sexual activity that is met with a good deal of repugnance even in today's tolerant attitude in the West.

It is safe to say that the majority of women find the thought of anal sex distasteful, but some females will go along with the practice to please their male partners.

There are though, those heterosexual couples whose preferred pleasure is anal sex. And, amongst those couples, it can often be the experienced, mature and sexually adventurous woman who expresses a preference for this form of sexual intercourse.

This subject now brings me to a letter that I received from a married man called John.

John wrote to tell me that he and his wife both enjoyed watching blue movies of couples having anal sex. He went on to say that, turned on by what they saw, they had tried anal intercourse. However, John's wife had found penetration too painful.

John wanted to know if hypnosis would help his wife to have further anal sex. I told him that I would not try hypnotherapy on his wife in order to change her mind. I would only help her if she wanted my guidance.

John gave me the impression of being a selfish lover; he needed to be told that the anus is very sensitive and prone to tearing.

I wondered if his wife really wanted to have sex this way, knowing that the majority of women are repulsed even by the thought of anal stimulation.

The advice that I decided to give John was that if his wife genuinely wanted to have anal sex then this could be achieved.

I told John that his wife could get used to anal penetration by practising with a vibrator purchased from a sex shop. She could graduate from a small to a larger sized vibrator over a period of time, and this device would help to stretch her anal muscles.

The other advice that I gave to John was the same that I give to any couples who have or want to have anal sex.

The woman should always empty her bowel before engaging in anal sex. This should be done either by a natural motion or with the aid of an enema.

For the reason of basic hygiene, the vagina should never be entered with the same condom that has been used for anal sex. If the same condom is used, this irresponsible action could give cystitis to a partner, or an even worse condition such as hepatitis or HIV. It cannot be stressed enough that the anal area is one of the most disease prone regions of the human body. Therefore, always have two condoms ready if relevant to your sexual activity.

The condom that is used for anal sex should be continually lubricated because the rectum absorbs lubricant very quickly. Use only water based products. Advice concerning lubricants is given with most condom packs so do read the instruction carefully.

Anal sex should be approached in a very gentle manner. The male partner should gently enter the anus. Once the head of the penis is inserted, stop for a few moments to help the anal muscles relax. Once this has been achieved the pace can be increased.

I shall end this chapter by saying that a key to sexual fulfilment is when both partners agree to what they want to introduce into their sex lives. This is what sexual compatibility is all about.

10

The Secret of Developing Breasts

The subject of cross-dressing, which I discuss in the chapter *The Secret Woman in Some Men's Lives - the Last Taboo*, reminded me of the e-mail that I received one day from George.

George explained to me that he had been cross-dressing for many years. However, he told me that he wanted to go beyond cross-dressing and have a sex change operation – and he wanted my advice.

George had seen his doctor about gender reassignment but the doctor had made him feel stupid, especially after referring him to a psychiatrist.

George was not at all happy about his doctor's lack of understanding or sympathy. Nor was he happy knowing that it would take years before he could have a gender change operation.

My enquirer wanted to start his gender transformation right away and he wanted to start by having female breasts.

George was a typical case of a pre operation transsexual who felt extremely frustrated at being faced with a waiting period before being able to have gender reassignment.

I suggested that he consult a private specialist because he would then be able to bypass the two year waiting period recommended by the UK National Health Service.

George did not respond to that idea because of the thousands of pounds it would cost for private treatment.

I then suggested that he could try taking certain herbs that have been known to enlarge women's breasts. I pointed out that I could give no guarantee that they would work. George said, "It's worth giving the herbs a try."

These are the two herbs that I mentioned to George:

Fenugreek (*Trigonella foenum-graecum*)

This plant's seeds contain diosgenin, a chemical compound that produces the female hormone estrogen (oestrogen in the USA). The effect of this hormone on the body is breast enlargement.

Fennel (*foeniculum vulgare*)

Fennel is another estrogenic herb.

The story of George was typical of the transsexual who feels trapped in the wrong body and wants to change gender.

The transsexual's need for gender reassignment is compelling, and can lead to suicide if that need is not satisfied.

Transsexuals are commonly referred to in the male gender because the majority of transsexuals are male to female. In comparison, there are far less female to male transsexuals.

There have been some high profile transsexuals through the years including the beautiful male to female Caroline Cossey who was a Bond girl in one of the James Bond movies.

In the UK the *Beaumont Society* and the *Gender Trust* support and help transsexuals. Both of these respected organizations are listed with contact details in the *Miscellaneous Information* section.

11
Who's a Big Baby?

It is, to say the least, an understatement for me to comment that my work is never run of the mill or boring. This fact has been brought home time and again but some of my "stranger than fiction" cases are even stranger than others. The following story is a perfect example.

From out of the blue a man turned up one day with one of the most extraordinary requests ever. His name was David and he wanted me to make him a special hypnosis tape. The tape that he wanted me to create was to be one that would make him wet his bed.

David told me after an introductory chat that he was an adult baby who, although often fulfilling his fantasy with his "nana" Jane and "mummy" Jill, had "progressed". It was now his desire to wet his nappy – in his bed – every night. He told me that being an adult baby was very rewarding and that the thought of reversing his toilet training was even more stimulating. He had heard about hypnosis tapes being used to turn adult babies back to pre toilet training bed wetters.

I arranged for David to have a full consultation with me for the following week and at the appointed time my client arrived looking very smart in a navy pinstripe suit.

David told me that he was a medical salesman who travelled throughout the UK and that he was regarded by his colleagues as even-tempered and stable, although that was not how he felt.

David said, "For many years being an adult baby has given me a tremendous feeling of comfort and safety."

My client explained that his emotional and physical needs were catered for by role players such as nana Jane and mummy Jill. These two ladies of course were not fulfilling such roles out of the kindness of their hearts but were professional women catering to adult babies.

Nana Jane, I learned from my client, had an adult nursery in Brighton. She had a two-year old child of her own but was also a wet nurse to a number of adult babies.

David told me, "I loved sucking on her breast and feeding off her warm milk; it was sensational. After she had fed me she would rub my back, change my nappy, put my dummy in my mouth and sing me to sleep until I closed my eyes. But now I want to totally fulfil my fantasy and wet the bed at night."

Many adult babies are particularly stimulated by reversing their toilet training. This is what my client wanted to do and it would be in this area that my hypnosis tape would help him. The reality is of course that many who revert to their pre toilet training phase lose all control of their bowel movements.

Toilet training started when we were first taught to control our bodily functions. This programming can also be seen as a symbol of denial for our physical and emotional feelings, so we learned at an early age that the adult world expected us to inhibit our urge to taste, touch, feel and smell everything in our surroundings.

The phenomenon of adults who want to revert to babyhood, known as *paraphilic infantilism*, is really in a unique category of its own.

There is nothing overtly sexual in the adult baby scenario, but those who want to act out their infant role fantasies do so with those prostitutes who provide a nanny and mummy service. There are also those who specialize exclusively in running a nursery for adult babies.

Whilst looking through my file for this chapter, I heard from a very reliable source that some years ago in rural Kent, such a service was being provided in the quiet market town of Faversham, a centre known for its famous Shepherd Neame beer, its annual *Faversham Hop Festival* - and where Bob Geldof has his country home.

In this tourists' idyllic Garden of England setting, this specialized service was attracting its own visitors - adult babies from London who would spend the weekend being pushed in prams in a more private garden of England, hidden behind the high walls of a local residence.

So, with no overt sexual activity involved in infantilism, and that includes paedophilia, you may well ask what need is satisfied.

The need to revert to infancy is the adult baby's way of dealing with anxiety and worry brought on by the pressures of everyday life. His regression allows him to shed the strain of being a grown-up in a stressful world by being an infant with a pretend mummy or nanny to look after his every need. He is going back to a period when a real mother and maybe a nanny too were on hand to look after him emotionally as well as physically. It was a time of innocence when he could do what he wanted to do and it did not matter what that was.

The adult baby's need to revert to infancy will involve dressing in outsize nappies and baby clothes, having a dummy to suck and often shaving off bodily hair. From time to time he may also change his baby boy role and adopt a baby girl role because gender switching can also be part of the fantasy scenario.

The mummy or nanny role player who is an integral part of the game will bath her adult baby, rub his back as if to bring up wind, talk in "coochy coo" baby language and involve her charge in tiny tot games.

If all this sounds like the profile of a very inadequate or dysfunctional personality, let me say that many adult babies are highly intelligent, successful, professional people such as solicitors, judges, doctors and senior civil servants.

For many of us, communicating anger, sadness, love and enjoying the release of a good belly laugh, can be hard in adult life. We become inhibited in the way we express ourselves, so we erect emotional and social barriers, whereas the adult baby - who does not want to be in control - is not restricted and explores and releases his emotions.

The adult baby is doing in his own way what many of us would like to do too…

Letting it all hang out

So what about the sexual make-up of the adult baby?

You will have seen with David, who was a typical case, that there was no apparent sexual motivation involved in his role playing, just a strong and dominating mother fixation.

"Dominating" and "mother" are keys to the adult baby's sexual make-up. He is attracted to dominant and maternal figures like matrons, senior hospital nurses, female doctors, headmistresses and of course nannies. He will also be sexually turned on by big breasted females.

His attraction to dominant mother figures, which does not surface overtly when he is baby role playing, but is part of his adult sex drive, will find expression with a sexually dominant partner with whom he can be sexually submissive.

Most adult babies have had past lives as children in orphanages, workhouses - or some institution where they relied on women for their maternal needs, and in many cases for their survival.

The way that such an experience - a strong imprint on the soul - can so often transform and manifest in a current life is that the person concerned will be sexually attracted to a dominant, maternal woman.

A couple of months after David had seen me he telephoned to say that my tape had worked for him perfectly.

David was one of many who make up the shadowy world of the adult baby devotees. From time to time one may get a hint of their activities when adult baby clothes are sold alongside fetish wear on the internet.

With the mother image central to this chapter, I shall end here with an appropriate anecdote about two of Hollywood's stars of yesteryear.

The beautiful actress Ava Gardner had several husbands, one of whom was actor-comedian Mickey Rooney, an extrovert character who was physically quite short. They made an odd looking couple because Mickey's lack of height was very noticeable when he was walking alongside the tall Ava.

Their marriage was regarded by many of the Hollywood community as a strange mismatch, but what was regarded as somewhat stranger, even by Hollywood standards, was that Mickey called Ava *mummy*, or as they say in America – *mommy*.

12

Too Much Masturbation

On a Wednesday morning one summer I turned on my computer so that I could go through my daily routine of reading e-mails. The first e-mail that I opened was from a woman called Geraldine.

In her letter she told me she had a problem - her husband Alan was more excited by masturbating and watching her have sex with his friend than making love to her.

I e-mailed a reply to Geraldine and an appointment was made for her and her husband to come and see me for a consultation on the following Tuesday.

On the Tuesday morning only Geraldine arrived for the appointment. Alan had lost his nerve and decided not to put in an appearance.

Geraldine was about 5' 5" in height. It was hard to tell her age but I would have put her in her late forties. She had short cropped brown hair and a very good figure. I learned later that she had been a photographic model.

I took Geraldine through to my consultation room, promptly reassuring her because I could see from her flushed face that she was very embarrassed about the prospect of discussing a personal marital problem.

I told my client that I had covered just about every sexual problem that existed and there was nothing she could say that would shock me. I added that I thought she was very brave to come and see me alone.

This woman was in need of help and the last thing she needed was to feel uncomfortable.

After putting Geraldine at ease, I asked her to give me the history of her relationship with her husband.

My client told me that she and Alan had been married for twenty-five years, that they were virgins on their wedding night – and that the wedding night had been a disaster. She described how Alan had twice tried to make love to her but without success. He had fumbled and "jerked about" and on both occasions penetrated her anus. This had hurt terribly and she had screamed out.

Geraldine told me, "When he gave up trying to penetrate me, he knelt at the side of me and masturbated until he came over my breast. We had no idea of foreplay at all at that time. After the honeymoon Alan continued to masturbate in this manner. It was a long time before we actually had full intercourse. I was very disappointed with intercourse.

Ninety-nine percent of our sex life was masturbation on both sides. We progressed to oral sex and the first time Alan came in my mouth I was surprised how nice it felt and tasted."

Geraldine then went on to tell me that over the last couple of years there had been a change in Alan's sexual routine because he had become sexually turned on by what she described as "absolutely filthy" talk whilst he masturbated over her. My client told me that she hated the dirty talking and it was turning her off sex.

"Have you told him this Geraldine?" I asked.

"Yes, over and over again but he's not listening or doesn't care. We also take chances having oral sex in car parks such as supermarket and council car parks. These places are not safe and we could easily be caught. But this seems to turn us on. Lately Alan and I have found some lovely places in woods and countryside which are very secluded. Alan has now started to take photos of me naked. On one of these visits while we were lying on the grass and Alan was masturbating over my breast, he said to me, 'You know, Roger really fancies you. He said he would love to fuck you.'"

I asked Geraldine who Roger was and she told me that he was a friend of Alan's.

My client then continued, "Alan also told me that Roger had not been circumcised. Never having been with any other partner, the thought of being with a man with a foreskin really turned me on. Alan is circumcised and he always says a man with a foreskin gets more pleasure from sex because of the skin rubbing up and down the penis. Also, Alan says that a woman gets more pleasure from giving oral [sex] to a man with a foreskin. This is because the woman would feel the skin rubbing in and out of her mouth. So, after giving this some thought, this started to excite me. It was agreed Alan would arrange it with his friend to come with us on our next photo shoot.

On our next photo shoot Roger came with us.

We stopped at our usual place and walked across the field to our part of the woods. Once there I started to undress.

I could see Roger looking at my body and this excited me. Alan started taking photos of me in various positions. It was apparent that Roger had an erection. Alan whispered to me, 'Shout Roger over and ask him if he wants his photo taken with you.' I waved Roger over and before we knew it, I was undoing his zip. Then I took out his penis and it looked wonderful. The first thing I did was to rub it up and down, just to see the skin moving up and down. Next I put it in my mouth and Roger [ejaculated] within seconds, all over my mouth and face. He did not stop coming for [a long] time. He told me [he] had dreamt of this moment all week since Alan had asked him to join us."

Geraldine told me that the three of them had continued with this scenario for the last eighteen months. The problem was that Roger had recently remarried and she felt that sex with him should now stop, feeling that it was wrong to encourage Roger to cheat on his wife. Alan though was insisting that their group sex sessions continued.

When Geraldine's consultation was over we arranged a time and date for her husband Alan to come and see me. Geraldine assured me that she would do everything she could to make sure that Alan kept the new appointment.

The day arrived for Alan's consultation and I was pleased when my doorbell rang at the appropriate time.

I opened the door to see standing before me a small, thin man with a receding hairline. Alan introduced himself and I took him through to my therapy room where I sat him down.

As we began talking, I could tell that he was nervous. Like Geraldine before him, I put Alan at ease by assuring him that I was used to dealing with every kind of sexual problem.

I gently instructed him to tell me about his relationship with Geraldine.

Alan began by telling me that he loved Geraldine who he had met when she was a topless photographic model and he was a photographer.

"I did many photo shoots with various topless models," he told me. "This always turned me on and I would masturbate over the photos."

"Why did you do this Alan?"

"I had a very strict upbringing by my parents. They were big churchgoers and up until the age of twenty-one and above I had to be in by 9 pm. For me girls were a no-no. Sex was evil and never to be talked about. This was when I got into masturbation. It was just me in my bedroom with my magazines of naked women. I would masturbate morning and evening over the photos. This made me feel powerful as I could masturbate over any beautiful woman I wanted."

Whilst Alan was talking to me, I realized that he was more into power and control than balanced sex.

I asked him to tell me what, apart from masturbation or any other sexual activity, made him feel powerful.

He thought about my question for awhile and then told me that being a professional photographer had made him feel powerful.

Alan qualified his answer by saying, "Having beautiful women taking off their clothes in front of me. They needed me. I had the power to make or break them. This turned me on and I had great satisfaction masturbating over their photos."

"How long did you continue to be a photographer after meeting Geraldine?" I asked.

"About six months. She started to get jealous over some of the girls and the hours I was working."

"So what kind of work did you do next?" I queried.

"I was a manager for a mobile phone company but I lost my job when I developed an ear problem."

"How did that make you feel Alan?" I probed.

"Angry, very angry. I had worked all hours under the sun for this company. Then as soon as my hearing problem started they got rid of me."

"What are you doing now Alan?"

"I work shifts in a parcel sorting warehouse for a transport company. Sorting out parcels for destinations throughout the UK."

"Now tell me about your childhood Alan."

My client told me that he had had a very strict Catholic upbringing. He was an only child who never felt wanted. When he went to school he was bullied because he was small. His parents had not been sympathetic about the bullying and had told him to stand on his own feet. His friends were never allowed to visit him at home and up until the age of fifteen he had to be in the house by 6.30 in the evening. As Alan had mentioned earlier, sex was thought of as evil and the subject was taboo. He was never told the facts of life by his parents and all he knew about sex was what he read in his erotic magazines. Having adult literature in his bedroom without his parents' knowledge made him feel good. He finally left home when he was twenty-three years old.

When the consultation came to a close we talked afterward for a time and I explained to Alan that it was a myth that men with foreskins had better sex than those who had been circumcised. I also made it quite clear to him that normal masturbation is fine (read the chapter *Pleasuring Your Sexual Self*). Abnormal, that is, obsessive masturbation, is not. I told Alan that in my opinion his masturbating had become an obsession. I warned him that too much could affect his hormone level. I added that a medical research programme had been conducted that had found a link between hair loss and excessive masturbation.

I pointed out to Alan that by cutting down on masturbating and reducing his number of ejaculations, his body would be able to replenish itself of lost nutrients and hormones.

I tactfully told Alan that I thought he was too much into control because he had orchestrated everything in his sex life with Geraldine, even down to Roger having sex with his wife. I also gently asked him to think about whether he was hiding any gay feelings.

Summing up, I told my client that it was not up to me to tell him and his wife how to conduct their sex lives but they should know they were missing out by not having normal sexual intercourse.

I also advised Alan that his upbringing was responsible for his sexual behaviour.

I created and gave Alan a magickal burner oil to help him stop his excessive masturbation.

To date both Alan and Geraldine are having healing with me. I give them reiki healing and distant healing to help them achieve a more balanced and rewarding sex life together.

For those of you who wish to break the habit of excessive masturbation, any of the following essential oils should help you:

- **Marjoram wild** *(Origanum vulgare)*
- **Thyme red** *(Thymus vulgaris)*
- **Ginseng Siberian** *(Eleutherococcus senticosus)*

Put between five and ten drops of oil in a burner and then add water to disperse the oil before heating.

When burning essential oils for the purpose of healing, it is necessary to take yourself off to your own private space and meditate on the healing which you wish to take place. As you do so, be conscious of the aroma and spiritual vibrations given off by the oil that you are burning. This procedure can be likened to burning incense to induce an altered state of consciousness for the purpose of spell-working or for conducting witchcraft rituals.

Please observe the usual precautions when heating oils with a naked flame and make sure there are no flammable objects nearby that can catch fire.

For a brief but concise explanation of reiki and some of the other subjects covered or mentioned in this book, I refer you to Belinda Whitworth's excellent book *New Age Encyclopaedia.*

Section 3
Past Life Regressions

1
Captain of the Guards

L iz was a lesbian who was in a very happy gay relationship yet she had constant headaches which caused problems with her sex life.

Before she came to see me, Liz had had a full medical examination. Her doctor could find nothing physically wrong with her. An allergy test failed to reveal anything either.

Liz had read a newspaper article about certain illnesses being cured by alternative healing, including hypnosis. She gave the subject of complementary medicine some thought and decided to consult me.

Liz, a well educated woman, had been working as a solicitor for the past seven years. She enjoyed her work immensely. However, the constant headaches, which she said started in her neck, were getting too frequent for her liking.

When she came to see me I suggested hypnotic regression. She responded by saying that she felt that her headaches, "may have nothing to do with a past life", but she was desperate and willing to try anything that might provide a cure.

I soon put Liz into a hypnotic state and took her back in time. It was not long before she returned to a former life as a man.

In this past life, Liz was Charles. The significant stage of the regression came when Liz as Charles, was a thirty-five year old captain of the guards in England.

Charles told me that the civil war in England was under way and that he was preparing his men for battle. He said that he was, "a very unhappy man." Unmarried, he expressed the feeling that he had achieved little of great importance in his life and then said, "I am getting so tired of all the fighting."

Throughout the regression, Charles kept complaining about the "heavy metal helmet" that he was wearing. He told me that his head armour was wearing him down.

Carrying on with the regression, I asked Charles where he was.

He replied, "In a market town somewhere near Yeominster. I am taking my men into battle and it's senseless. Killing is wrong."

"Have you always been in the army?" I queried.

Charles answered, "For most of my life. It was good at first but I am tired of this life. I would have liked to have married if my work had been different."

I noticed that while Charles was talking he was moving his head as if the heavy metal helmet was still bothering him.

I asked Charles to move on and tell me what happened next.

He responded with, "I have to lead my men into battle for more pointless killing. There are swords swinging and blood everywhere. I hate having to lead my men to their deaths."

Suddenly my client gave a scream of agony and I asked what was wrong." Charles cried out, "My arm has been hit. I've fallen to the ground. The pain is excruciating. A soldier hit out with his sword and sliced through the top of my arm near my neck. Most of my left arm is hanging off. Blood is all around me and I feel so strange."

Giving me no time at all to ask Charles what he meant by his comment of feeling "strange", I saw that my client was hardly breathing and seemed to be drifting away.

For a few seconds I was worried, but then to my great surprise, my client's face took on a beautiful glow.

"What is happening to you Charles?"

In a calm voice he answered, "I can see a light. It's drawing me closer and closer. The more I move closer to the light, the more my pain is easing."

I instructed Charles to continue to tell me what was happening to him.

"I died a very slow and painful death. My body was in such agony before the spirit beings came to me. They took me through a long golden tunnel. It was so beautiful."

That was the end of Liz's regression which she had found a truly spiritual experience. She was amazed that she had carried her pain through from her life as Charles to her present incarnation. She realized though, through the insight gained by her regression that she was "echoing" the severe sword wound near her neck, combined with the uncomfortable weight of the protective helmet that she had suffered in her previous life. Those experiences materialized as a headache in Liz's present life – and explained why her headaches always started in the neck.

In many cases, unaccountable health conditions can be traced back to an incident in a past life. This does not mean that you should not consult a doctor or medical specialist when you have an ongoing health problem. Please do so, but keep in mind that there could be a past life explanation for what ails you.

2

Why Childless?

Over the years I have met many interesting people who have come to me for help. Most of these folk never thought of themselves as unique individuals, not realizing that many diverse past life experiences had brought them to the present to give them their very own physical and spiritual identities. Most of my clients have no idea that their current circumstances and influences have past life connections.

Using hypnosis more often than not as my treatment of choice, I have regressed clients so that they can travel back in time, review their former lives and pinpoint past situations that could be causing problems in the present.

Without wanting to sound immodest I have to say that some miraculous cures have taken place after some of my hypnotherapy treatments. Clients who had lived with psychological and physical problems before receiving hypnotherapy, started on the road to recovery from the time of their regressions with me.

With the unique experience of a past life review, my clients have been able to learn the reason for their "unexplained" illnesses. Phobias have been eliminated too, including a fear of flying – which is an awful anxiety to deal with for anyone who is terrified of going aloft in an aircraft.

The following account was brought to mind after watching a television programme about the notorious killer known as *Jack the Ripper*. There were aspects of the *Ripper* documentary that reminded me of a woman I treated several years ago.

Here is the story of Jean who was regressed to a past life – and through the insight she gained, was able to see why she had a health problem and a phobia in her present life.

Jean knocked on my front door on a chilly February day in 1991. I opened the door to see a shivering, frighteningly thin woman standing outside. I invited her in and asked her why she had come to see me.

The poor girl stood in my hall, twiddling nervously at the buttons on her coat before she said in a waif-like voice…

"I have an illness and a phobia. I have blocked fallopian tubes and cannot have children." Referring to her husband, she added, "This was a very big disappointment for us both." She then continued, "My phobia is with London."

Jean stood there in my hall with her head hanging low and tears streaming down her cheeks, so I asked her softly how the phobia manifested and affected her.

As Jean wiped the tears away, she replied, "Whenever I visit London I am overcome with fear. It's so bad that I start to shake from head to toe for no logical reason. It's so irrational, but I cannot stop it. I am overtaken with dread. It's like a dark, distant memory haunting me, challenging me to find the answer. It's crazy."

I could not help but notice how pale and drained Jean looked as she stood looking down at the floor. This poor woman was very troubled.

With a deep intake of breath that seemed to give her renewed strength, she continued, "I am here today to find a solution to my problem. I have no choice. You see my husband's just been promoted and we've got to move [to] within the London district. Somehow I've got to beat this phobia. Please help me," she pleaded.

"I will try to do my best," I said.

I took Jean through to my consultation room, asked her to take off her coat and shoes and settled her in my special chair. I gave her a few moments to compose herself before wrapping a blanket around her tiny body. It was essential to keep her warm while the treatment was in progress because hypnotherapy causes the body temperature to drop.

I started Jean's hypnosis session as soon as she was relaxed enough to proceed.

Within minutes she started to talk to me slowly, not in her gentle Welsh accent but in a broad cockney accent.

"Where are you Jean?"

Responding to my question, Jean answered, "It's the East End of London and I am a little girl. It looks so strange here, like pictures of the Victorian era."

At this point my client began to breathe quite quickly. Calming her, I waited for her to resume. After a moment or two she continued.

"I don't know how old I am but I am very small and have no shoes on my feet. I look very dirty and the brown ragged dress I am wearing itches."

I asked, "Are you alone? Is your mother with you?"

Jean answered, "There is no-one with me and I am standing alone in an alleyway. If I lean against the wall I can get some warmth. It's so cold here. The cobblestone is wet and slippery. I can see our door but my mother won't let me in. She says she's working. I am so cold, so very cold. Why can't I get warm?"

The physical discomfort that Jean was feeling was quite real to her. It is quite common for a hypnotized patient to bring through a discomfort that is being experienced from an altered time frame. This is the patient's reality as it was in a past life. Reliving an experience or experiences, some of which can be horrific, such as Liz went through in *Captain of the Guards* is in fact the start of a client's cure.

However, Jean's experience of feeling abnormally cold was puzzling but I would soon find out why this condition was exaggerated.

Trying to take her mind off being cold, I gently probed her for more information about her mother, "What kind of work does your mother do?"

Jean answered directly, "She is a prostitute. I hate it when men come to the house because I have to wait in the alleyway until they have gone."

"Does your mother know how unhappy you feel about her work?" I asked.

"Yes, she knows but says she's got no choice otherwise we would end up in the workhouse."

"Where is your father?" I probed.

Jean replied sharply with an angry look on her face, "I ain't got one."

Moving away from the subject of her father, I said, "Tell me what you can see in the alleyway. Describe it to me."

Jean told me, "There are other children here; some are quite big. We are all cold. None of us have shoes on. Some are trying to get warm like me. Others are playing with stones. There are dead rats on the path and I have to step over them to get to the wall. But I can see my front door from here."

I instructed my client to move to the time when she was permitted to go back home. I was not prepared for what came next.

Without warning Jean went into a bout of violent shaking. She sobbed hysterically for all she was worth.

"What is wrong? Tell me what you are seeing" I gently requested.

With terrified gulps, Jean blurted out, "I watched and waited for a very long time. It started to get dark and rainy, so I crept in through the back door. Everything was quiet but there was such a bad stink in there. I walked through the door into the main room and oh my goodness, there is so much blood. She's been torn open; there are bits of her around the room. Oh God, she is dead; help, help."

Jean's terrified screams filled the room for the next five minutes. As her screaming subsided I reassured her that it was alright to continue. I gently but firmly instructed her to view the scene from above, as an objective observer, and to erase all emotional attachment. I then directed her to move on, "Tell me all that happened after you cried out for help."

"I was screaming so loudly and did not notice the room filling up with officers. A strange woman took hold of my arm and dragged me out into the street. I could hear one of the policemen vomiting and another was saying that it was worse than the slaughterhouse down the street. I kept crying for my mother and I heard someone mention taking me to the workhouse, so I ran away, slipped right past them and kept on running."

"Where did you go?" I prompted.

In a stressed voice Jean said, "Back to the wall. I am trying to get some warmth. It's so cold here and I want my mother."

"I want you to go back in time for me," I requested. "Return to the alleyway. Go back before you found your mother. Watch the front door. Tell me who goes into the house and who leaves."

Jean told me, "My mother is inside with the gentleman. I met him before they sent me outside."

It struck me when Jean said "gentleman", that such a title in those days, would only have been used to describe a member of the aristocracy or someone who was obviously rich; so I asked my client to describe what this gentleman looked like.

"I did not have time to see him," said Jean, "my mother sent me out. I know he wore a large hat and carried a walking cane. It was black and he was wearing dark gloves."

My client could give me no further description of this man or his identity so there was no point in pursuing this line of questioning any further. I therefore asked her to move forward six hours and describe what was happening.

"I can see a tiny frozen body huddled against the wall in the alleyway. It's my body. The little feet are blue with cold. I think I am about five or six years of age. People are standing around it. I recognize the policeman. He is the one who went to the house. He looks sad."

"Do you feel sad?" I asked.

"Not any more. Things are fine now. My mother is with me and we are moving away from this awful place. This had been a terrible life, but mother says we won't have to go there again. She says we are going to a new home. It's wonderful and I am now so warm and happy."

There was a wondrous expression of joy and tranquillity across Jean's face.

Before bringing my client back to full consciousness, I instructed her subconscious mind to see her forthcoming move to London in a positive light, and to concentrate on the good things that her husband's promotion could bring. I also impressed upon her that she no longer existed in the Victorian period and would not be experiencing the hardships she once endured. I also asked her to imagine her blocked fallopian tubes clearing.

Apart from the hypnotherapy session, I gave Jean a meditation visualizing exercise which she could carry out on a daily basis. I also gave her some magick spells to help her become pregnant. However, I did tell my client that my spells would only help her if it was in her destiny to get pregnant.

Jean's recent past life experience had been that of an innocent child. Not being able to conceive in her present life was not a punishment for some past misdemeanour.

It may well have been that Jean had agreed between lives to go through a childless future life in order to have that kind of experience.

Let me qualify this explanation by saying that the majority of witches, and Spiritualists too, believe that we move through a series of lives in order to gain every conceivable kind of human experience.

I end here with two candle magick spells for those of you who wish to have children but are having difficulty conceiving:

Candle magick spell

A red candle is required for this spell. On the candle etch the Goddess name ISIS. While you etch the name on the candle visualize yourself as pregnant. Light your candle and see the flame as the light of a new life.

Meditate upon the candle flame for several minutes and then snuff out the candle and keep it to use the next day.

Repeat this spell daily until the candle has burned through.

Candle magick spell for Christians

A white candle is required for this spell. On the candle etch the name JEHOVAH.

Light your candle, meditate upon being pregnant for a few minutes and then recite psalms 102 and 103.

Repeat this ritual daily until the candle has burned through.

Always burn your candle in a safe area and never blow but snuff it out. When the candle has burned down, bury the stub in your garden or throw it into running water.

3

Sterility and the Past

Ian had seen his doctor, consulted a specialist and gone through all the tests to try and determine why he was sterile. At the end of the whole tiring procedure no-one was any the wiser.

It was Ian's wife Sandra who came to see me in the hope that I could solve the mystery of her husband's sterility. Like so many folk with personal problems, Sandra had come to see me as a last resort after all other professional avenues of enquiry had been exhausted.

I am obviously guided by a strong intuitive feel for a situation and my inner voice was telling me that the best route to take with this problem was to conduct a hypnotherapy session with my client Sandra.

I made sure that Sandra was quite comfortable and relaxed and then put her into a hypnotic state. I then asked her to go back to her previous life and tell me who she was and where she was.

My client told me that her name was Jane Cattone and she was sixteen years old and working on her father's land.

She then went on to say, "I work on the farm, sometimes milking our cow. Mostly I help my mother with the chores. I have a brother called Ben but he's not right."

Interrupting her, I asked her what she meant by her brother not being right. She told me that he had been brain damaged since his birth and he was now eleven years old.

Jane carried on without any prompting and told me that she planned to marry Tom, "a dark-haired good looking young man."

After she chattered on about matters of little significance I asked Jane to jump ahead a few years.

Moving forward in time Jane told me that she had married Tom in 1729 and they had their own smallholding. They were happy with life and although not very rich it did not matter to them. Moving ahead again Jane told me that she and Tom now had two children and their third was expected in June.

After talking about the birth to be of their third baby my client started clutching her stomach and moaning in pain. I could see beads of sweat on her face but I urged her to continue.

Jane continued, "My baby won't come; the pain is terrible. I am in childbirth but can't birth it."

I asked her if anyone was with her.

Between gasping with pain she told me, "My mother and Tom. They keep telling me to push the baby but still it won't come."

Go beyond the pain, I insisted.

In response she sobbed, "Oh my poor baby it's dead. I am also dead. My family are around me now and they are all weeping. I never wanted to leave them, my lovely children and my dear Tom."

Jane's spirit continued to stay with her family for a good while after her death. It took a lot of effort for her to move on.

When Jane came back to the present and became Sandra again, she told me that she understood how a spirit could become earthbound.

Sandra was one of the many women who had died in a previous life giving birth. Most of those who died in this way expressed such sadness and regret for leaving their children and husbands behind.

When we think about childbirth in past times it was highly dangerous. And this is where a past life affecting a present existence comes into play. Many of the husbands who suffered the loss of their wives in past lives have become gynaecologists and paediatricians in their current incarnations. I believe that this is a vocational calling that comes from the Goddess.

Obviously not every case of sterility can be linked to a past life tragedy but for some it is a direct past life link.

If we can just imagine a husband's pain at seeing his wife dying trying to give birth to their child, then we can imagine the degree of guilt that he must have felt, even if he was not to blame in any way.

I often say to my clients that the psychology of guilt is that it seeks punishment. One wonders how many sterile men today, at a deep soul level, carry the pain of seeing a wife dying when trying to give birth to a baby in a past life, a pain that later manifests physically to stop them having children.

4

Barbara's Experience
- Another Childless Case

Barbara was one of a group who had responded to my newspaper request in 1992 for volunteers who would be willing to be hypnotically regressed. I conducted two regressions with this volunteer and she was kind enough to write to me later and describe the hypnosis experiences from her perspective. Here are her two letters.

Barbara's first past life regression

"After hypnosis had taken over, I found myself in a past life. I know not which year, era or century. It must have been way back due to the clothes I was wearing.

I was just standing. There seemed to be nothing around me. I felt I was nothing. I was standing on what appeared to be hard ground, sort of a beaten track, where many feet had trodden. In fact there seemed to be nothing or no-one around me, just me. I felt nothing at first, just empty and dead. Then the name came to me. Nora. Was I Nora? I must have been.

I was wearing some kind of smock or loose garment made of coarse linen, sort of beige shade. I felt I was pregnant, about six months. But I felt nothing emotionally, a walking corpse perhaps. Then Tarona asked me to go back to where I had come from, as I appeared to be running away.

I appeared to be lost. In my state I was lost in a sea of rejection, and hurt. Then suddenly there was a big house, a mansion style place with tall gates and a long driveway. I was running away from the big house, from the master whose child I was carrying. It was he who had rejected me, and in running away I had tried to lose myself completely. I must have wandered for a long time, days and possibly weeks.

Then Tarona asked me to move about and find out where I was. I was just standing alone and felt nothing. I wanted to die. Perhaps I was already dead. Then I found myself walking down a road, to my left were two small cottages. Two women appeared and helped me into a house. It was a small place. I had to go down two or three steps into the room. It was neat, a little bit dark. I noticed a wooden dresser of some sort, and a plain table and two chairs. The women were very kind to me. They could have been sisters. They fussed around and I felt such warmth and relief to be somewhere comfortable.

Then Tarona asked me to go to the time of the birth. But there was no pain, no birth. So I could only conclude that I was having a child I did not want, probably because I had been rejected by the father. I had no desire to live. I was about twenty-five years old. I had no prospects, nothing to live for. So I died in that cottage more or less as soon as I arrived. Being rejected by a man who I foolishly thought loved me, my spirit was broken. I had not eaten for ages, so obviously, whatever the two ladies had done for me was too late. I saw one of them put a cover over me, then nothing."

Barbara's second regression

"I discovered myself sitting on a bench somewhere. I was wearing a longish skirt, but not ankle length. I was wearing a cardigan, this too was long. It was [a] coloured Fair Isle.

Tarona asked me what nationality I might be. I thought perhaps I might be Dutch because I was wearing a clog. There didn't appear to be two clogs. Then suddenly I realized it wasn't a clog, or one clog. It was an unsightly shoe on my left foot; a club foot. I felt myself to be about forty years old. I seemed to be a very contented person in spite of my disability but my foot used to hurt and ache a lot. The pain sometimes came with such force, so much so that I actually felt the pain in my regression.

I can recollect living in a nice ordinary kind of house in a quiet street.

Tarona asked what my name was. It came easy, Sylvia Moran. At this point I was in the house. I recall coming down the quiet street and into a living room. Tarona asked am I married and did I have a husband. I could not recall at first. I looked around this very familiar room and there it was; a photograph or picture of a man in uniform standing in pride of place on a sideboard or dresser.

Tarona asked me to move ahead. Several years passed and I was in a hospital bed. There were nurses around, one quite close. There was some kind of cage at the foot of the bed. Then I realized it was over my club foot. But I no longer had a foot. Had it been eaten away? I was obviously dying of gangrene or some such thing. There was no real agony, just a feeling of wanting to let go.

Tarona asked me how old I was. Had I married again? I think I was around forty-five years of age. No, I hadn't married again. Anyway, who would want me with my ugly foot. She then asked me to go to a few seconds before my death. Suddenly he was there. Just as I knew him before he was killed in some war or other. He was in full uniform. His name came so readily, it was George. I was in his arms, he was holding me. At last I was safe. I was crying, sobbing and smiling all at once, because I [had] found him again. I had become emotional in my regression and the tears were real."

Barbara has no children in her present incarnation. Her husband, who was sterile, died some years ago.

In Barbara's first past life regression she described a tragic experience when she was taken advantage of by the lord of the manor which resulted in her carrying his baby. In her present incarnation she had a husband who was sterile. Was this husband the original lord of the manor who made Nora pregnant? And was he sterile to balance off his past life behaviour according to the law of karma? In between these two lives she tells of losing a husband in a war. In none of these lives has she had a relationship with a man that has run its full course, nor in any of these three lives has she had a child.

There would seem to be an interesting but tragic pattern of karma being played out here. Hopefully this soul will soon be able to move on from the sadness that has surrounded her over her last three incarnations.

5

He Wanted to be the Woman He was Before

Peter's hypnotic regression began on a cold December day in 1992. When I answered my doorbell and opened the front door on that grey winter's day a fantastic looking man was standing in front of me. He had beautiful honey blonde hair which was long, straight and well groomed. He possessed deep blue eyes and the longest eyelashes I have ever seen. His features were perfectly formed and the only way to describe Peter was "drop dead gorgeous." However, his beauty was feminine rather than masculine.

Peter was very effeminate in his body movements and speech mannerisms and you did not have to be psychic to know that he was gay.

As soon as I started Peter's past life regression he returned to his conception. Let me say that a conception sequence had never ever happened before during any of my clients' regressions.

"It's all wrong, I don't want to be conceived," Peter said.

Puzzled, I asked, "Why not?"

"Because being born will mean I will become a male," he answered.

Not fully understanding what the problem was at this stage, I urged Peter to carry on and asked him to tell me what he was seeing.

Responding to my request to continue, he said, "I am in a bedroom and there is a brown mahogany wardrobe at the bottom of the bed. The bed is covered with a green candlewick bedspread."

The more Peter described the room and its contents for me, the more distressed he became. Peter had returned to the bedroom in which he had been conceived, and the recall of this room, and its significance for him, was making my client very agitated. I gently asked him to go back further in time.

Soon Peter was back in the eighteenth century where he said he was a "female called Sarah." He continued, "I am wearing a long dress and it feels very rough on my skin. It's 'itchy'."

As I observed Peter in his hypnotic state as Sarah, I could see that he was restless. He was obviously feeling irritated by the coarse cloth of the dress.

"Are you pretty?" I probed.

"Jack thinks so", he giggled.

"Who is Jack?" I asked.

"He is my future husband, Sarah answered.

"What does Jack do; what sort of work does he do?" I enquired.

"Jack works with horses on the farm," Sarah responded.

"Do you work?" I queried.

"Yes," said Sarah, "I am a milkmaid."

I then requested Sarah to describe herself.

"My hair is very long and fair." Then after a pause she continued, "I am seventeen years old. Jack and I marry when I am eighteen. We were able to get an afternoon off work. We married in a little church used by the workers and servants alike."

Sarah told me that she and her husband were living somewhere in the Devon area, not too many miles from a castle. She then continued ...

"I love Jack very much and we are very happy together. My Jack is very handsome."

I could see a smile cross Peter's lips, who as Sarah, was describing happy times. Then without any warning my client burst into tears.

"Whatever is wrong Sarah? Please tell me," I pleaded.

"It's my Jack, there's been a bad accident and he's been killed," said Sarah.

It was difficult to understand what Sarah was saying because of her uncontrollable crying. Eventually, with my prompting, she moved on one year after the disaster.

Sarah told me about the accident that caused her husband Jack's death. She told me that he had been working with the horses when one of the animals had reared up after being stung by a bee. The rearing horse knocked Jack to the ground and then the animal trampled him to death.

Not wanting my client to feel any more stress, I instructed Sarah to move ahead to just five minutes after her own death.

"What do you see now?" I asked.

"The body of a thin young woman," was my client's reply.

"Was she alone when she died?" I prompted.

"Yes."

I continued with my questioning. "In the short time you were married to Jack, did you have any children?"

"No, Jack died a few months after we were married. We both wanted to have children and if he'd not died so soon we would have had them," was the answer.

"Looking back on your life as Sarah," I asked, "what was the lesson you learned from that life?"

"It had been a short marriage – but a good one. I loved being a woman and having such a strong man as Jack to hold me in his arms," responded my client.

While still under hypnosis, I asked Peter if he had met Jack in his present life.

"Yes, I have," he said, "but there can be no possible chance of a relationship between us this time."

"Why is that?" I queried.

"Because," said Peter, "Jack is a straight man and I am trapped in this man's body. Now you understand why I did not want to be conceived in the first place. It was a mistake for me to come back as a male this time. I should have been female and could have married Jack and had a proper life again."

I brought Peter out of his regression and then we talked for awhile.

I told my client that his present life was not a mistake and that there must be some divine plan for him.

I added that although his sexuality and gender were different in his present incarnation, he was still on a spiritual path. I pointed out that mistakes are never made about the gender role that we have in our various lives. To emphasize the point that I was making, I told Peter that he had incarnated as a male for a specific purpose and that if he searched inwardly, he would find out why this was so.

From my perspective as a psychotherapist, Peter's past life link with his present incarnation had not only been unusual and interesting, but the regression had pinpointed his frustration at being male and homosexual.

This particular case is not meant to imply that all gay men and women are unhappy with their sexuality or gender because we all have a different set of past and present life circumstances.

We are here to live many lives, lived as male and female, gay and heterosexual, rich and poor, healthy and disabled, experiencing every kind of human condition so that we can progress along the spiritual path.

In conclusion, I recommend a trilogy of books that deal with the subjects of reincarnation and the purpose of life. These three volumes, by American author Chelsea Quinn Yarbro, are *Messages from Michael, More Messages from Michael* and *Michael's People.*

6
The
Paedophile

Even as a sex witch, I am sometimes faced with certain aspects of human sexual behaviour that I would prefer not to deal with. In that respect I am no different from the majority of human beings.

Over the years I have helped so many who have had every kind of sexual problem. But, until an evening in 1990, I had never been approached by a paedophile.

It was about six o'clock on a cold Monday evening when my telephone rang. I picked up the telephone and heard a well spoken male voice at the other end of the line. Without any preliminary small talk, the man immediately started pleading with me to help him.

He told me quickly and honestly that he was a paedophile. Without pausing, he went on to tell me that he could remember parts of his former life and these glimpses of a past existence were arousing him sexually. He told me that he wanted to stop these feelings and live a normal life.

I knew that I had to see this man, even though paedophiles sicken me. I arranged an appointment for my caller and within a few days he was sitting before me in my home.

Terrance was a tall, well dressed man. He had dark brown wavy hair and deep, penetrating blue eyes. He told me that he was thirty-one years old. However, when I asked him for his home address and telephone number he refused to divulge this information.

My deeply rooted prejudice against paedophiles was making me feel uncomfortable about his close presence. I knew though that I had to ignore my prejudice and be objective if I was going to stop this man from hurting children. The only way to deal with this situation would be to help the person who was now sitting opposite me.

Terrance's voice interrupted my thoughts as he said, "All my life I've had flashbacks and dreams. I keep seeing this little girl and this image gives me an erection. My wife is getting suspicious. She thinks I am having an affair."

Surprised that my client was married, I asked him, "How long have you been married?"

"Six years," Terrance replied.

"Have you got any children Terrance?" I asked.

"Not yet, but we are planning to have some," he answered.

I decided to carry out a hypnotic regression there and then. Normally, another appointment would have been made, but I thought that I dare not let this man go. Here was this potentially dangerous stranger sitting in front of me and I did not have his address or telephone number. There was no way to trace him. It would have been far too risky to let him wait for another appointment. I just could not let this man vanish into the night.

Thankfully, Terrance agreed to a regression.

I put my client into a hypnotic state and I was soon guiding him back in time to a former life. I instructed him to tell me all about what he was seeing, feeling and doing.

Terrance told me, "I am standing in front of a fire. It's [in] a big dark room. The curtains are dark and I'm not wearing any clothes. I am a female called Emily."

"How old are you Emily?" I enquired.

"Nine years old," responded my client before continuing, "There is a man in this room and he is looking at my naked body."

---

* In Victorian times prostitutes were often referred to as "dolly mops" and this may be why Emily called her vagina a dolly.

I broke in at this point and asked, "Does your mother know this man's in the room?"

Terrance replied, "Yes, she's brought him to look at me. She brings many men to look at me."

"Do they only look at your body Emily?" I queried.

"No, they do other things."

"What other things do they do? Tell me all that you experience in this room," I prompted.

My client continued, "I am told to lie down and open my legs wide so the men can see inside my dolly.* Some of them put their fingers inside me, others put their face down there and put their tongue around and inside me. Some try to push their fingers up my bum but it hurts and I don't like it. Some of the men put their willy in my mouth and I am told to lick it. Also, I am told to suck the round things at the bottom of their willy. I have to keep doing this until the stuff comes out of the man's willy."

In the above sequence, Emily was obviously referring to the men's penises, testicles and ejaculation.

Carrying on with the regression, I asked Emily to move on a little in time and tell me what had been happening to her.

Emily then recounted the following shocking experience up to the time of her death.

"A man with a big red beard knelt down on the floor and looked at my dolly. He pushed his finger inside me before walking over to my mother. He whispered to her and she looked over at me and then quietly spoke to the man. He put his hand in his pocket and pulled out a pouch. I could see him giving my mother more money. She then walked over to me and tied my hands to the bedstead with a couple of her old stockings.

This had never happened to me before and I was very frightened. I shouted to my mother, asking her why she had done this to me. She told me to shut up because the man had paid good money for this. Next, the man stood at the bottom of the bed and undid a big belt that held his pants up.

When the man rolled off me he put his pants on and walked out. My mother came over to me and untied my hands. When I looked down, I could see blood around my dolly and down my legs. My mother threw a wet cloth at me and told me to clean myself up.

After this time, all the men who came to our room paid money to my mother and they had full sex with me.

After about the third time I stopped feeling any pain.

When I was twelve years old my mother sold me to a brothel and it was in this brothel I became pregnant for the first time.

I was in great pain and the labour was long. After the birth the baby was taken out of the room. They told me the baby was dead.

At the age of fifteen years I was sold to a middle-aged man. He took me to his home in Bristol. I was his property in all respects. I died giving birth to his child at sixteen years of age."

"How did you feel about dying in this way?" I asked.

Still talking as Emily, my client replied, "Happy, it was a life of depravation."

Before terminating the regression, I instructed my client that from that day forward, he should cease having any form of sexual or abnormal interest in children.

After I brought Terrance out of the regression we talked for a time. I was alarmed when he told me that, during the hypnotic regression, he had an erection as he was reliving the sexual encounters he had as Emily.

I asked my client to promise to contact me again in a couple of weeks to let me know if he had experienced any changes taking place, both when awake – and when asleep. He agreed to do this and he also asked me to perform some spells for him.

Terrance wanted some magick spells to overcome his unclean thoughts about children and he wanted to have balance and peace. My client was a Christian and asked me if I could perform some spells that were in keeping with his beliefs. I told him that spells performed with psalms were very effective. However, I pointed out that in addition to my spell casting on his behalf, he would also have to carry out the same spells. He agreed to do this.

The spells that were performed, combining candle magick and Christian psalms, are given below:

Spell one:
To overcome unclean thoughts

Take a purple candle and anoint it with olive oil in the following manner: Apply some oil to the middle of one side. Now rub the oil down to the bottom of the candle. Then place a dab of oil on the same centre spot and rub it up to the top of the candle.

Now light your candle and recite psalms sixty-nine and seventy.

After reciting the two psalms, snuff out the candle. Do not extinguish the candle by blowing it out because the spell will not work if you do so. Extinguish by using a candle snuffer or an old spoon.

Repeat this spell once a day until the candle burns down. When you have no more than a candle stub, bury the end in the garden or throw the small remainder into running water.

Spell two:
To achieve self-balance

Take a purple candle and anoint it with olive oil in the following manner: Apply some oil to the bottom of the candle on one side. Next, rub the oil up to the middle of the candle and stop there. Now apply oil at the top of the candle and rub it downward, stopping at the same centre spot that you reached before in the middle of the candle.

Now light your candle and recite psalms one hundred and twelve and one hundred and thirteen.

After reciting the two psalms, snuff out the candle in the same way as described with the first spell.

Repeat this spell once a day and follow the same procedure for the disposal of the candle stub as described in Spell One.

Section 4
Advice

1
Erection Problems

If a man is unable to get or sustain an erection, it is very distressing, not only for the man but for his partner too. As a sex witch, I am contacted at least a dozen times a week by men seeking my help for this unhappy situation.

One of the most worrying aspects of this setback to sexual harmony is that this condition is on the increase, hence the high sales of the drug Viagra.

It is my personal belief that many individuals have become very out of tune with the universe, consequently losing touch with their higher, spiritual selves. They have, as a result of becoming disconnected, alienated themselves from the magickal pleasures that have been given to us as our birthright by the Gods and Goddesses.

One of the most important of the magickal pleasures is sex. If there is any imbalance in the spiritual, emotional or material life of the person concerned, then as sure as night follows day, that person's sex life will suffer.

At any first counselling session when my client has an impotence problem, I ask about the lifestyle of the man or couple concerned. This question is very important because more often than not, men will confess to hating their jobs and the excessively long hours they work in order to keep their women happy. Men will often confide to me that their partners have become materialistic monsters.

With such a disharmonious domestic situation, it should come as no surprise to the woman that all her man wants to do in bed is sleep, or if sexual intercourse is attempted, he is unable to get or maintain an erection.

Another reason for the man's impotence could be that his chakras are blocked. Chakras are spinning wheels of energy that connect us to our soul and to the universe.

There are seven main chakra points in the human body. They are:

* **Base** (base of spine/groin area)
* **Sacral** (below the navel)
* **Solar plexus** (above the navel)
* **Heart** (chest)
* **Throat** (base of the neck)
* **Centre of forehead** (the third eye/psychic sight)
* **Crown** (top of the head)

The following seven chakra exercise is designed to clear away emotional debris. Not only is this exercise beneficial to sexually stressed men but it is also a good ritual for women with low libidos.

Find a comfortable chair and sit in it with your bare feet firmly on the ground. Keep your back straight.

Give yourself time to assume a relaxed state of mind, then visualize a bright red ball of energy appearing at the base of your spine. See this red sphere spinning in a clockwise direction. Always visualize the spheres spinning clockwise throughout the whole chakra exercise. Now breathe in and draw the red ball of energy up to your sacral chakra which is below your navel.

As you draw the red ball up to your sacral region, see the sphere change colour and become orange. At the same time visualize the orange sphere stimulating your pelvic region, then breathe out.

Next breathe in. As you do so, see your solar plexus chakra become a spinning ball of yellow. As you visualize the spinning yellow sphere, feel emotional peace and breathe out.

Follow-up by breathing in and sense the yellow ball moving to your heart chakra and transforming into a pink sphere of pulsating energy. Feel this pink energy filling you with love and compassion – and breathe out.

Now breathe in and sense the pink sphere moving to your throat chakra where you see it turn into a blue ball. Breathe out when the blue sphere reaches your throat.

Breathe in as you see the blue ball moving to your third eye chakra where the sphere turns purple. At this stage, because you have reached your psychic centre, you may become aware of the cause of your erection problem. Now breathe out as you move the purple ball of spinning energy up to your crown chakra.

Breathing calmly, visualize the purple sphere of spinning energy turning white as it moves down your seven chakras. Feel this white ball purifying and cleansing away all your past negative emotions as it makes its way back to your base chakra.

Continue to breathe in and out calmly, totally relaxing, as you would in a meditation exercise after completing a series of yoga postures.

If the seven chakra exercise has had no effect on you, it is time to look at the attitude and habits of your female partner. During my work as a sex witch, my clients confide to me constantly about the relationship problems that inhibit their sex lives. I shall now share their disclosures with you.

Detailed here, with many of my own comments, are the main problems that are mentioned to me time and again:

The woman who makes critical remarks when her man expresses his sexuality. This type of female has a "Let's get it over with quickly" attitude.

The woman who, inhibited perhaps by a strict religious upbringing, has a feeling of guilt about sex.

The woman who believes that sex is only for making babies.

The woman taught from an early age that she must suppress her sexuality or be thought of as a "loose" female.

The woman who makes her man feel responsible for her having an orgasm - or not having one.

Never make a man feel responsible for you reaching a climax. If your man is at fault with his technique, just tell him what you like, or do not like, when having sex.

We often hear women complaining about being regarded as sex objects. Well, hello ladies; many men worry that they are **not** regarded as sex objects. If you show no physical interest in your man, then he may worry that there is something wrong with his body. Just remember, men are sensitive too.

With the above-mentioned in mind, remember to make love to all your man's body in the same way that you want him to make love to you. If you lie there like a corpse during sexual activity, you will make your man feel completely useless. Become totally familiar with your man's penis. Do not just hold it and give it a few quick strokes. Ask yourself how you would feel if your partner just grabbed your breasts or gave your vagina half a dozen hurried rubs. Would you be sexually stimulated by such treatment? I think not. Worship your man's wonderful tool and think of the pleasure that it can give you.

Talking at intimate moments about decorating the kitchen or the annual vacation will distract your man from experiencing the full pleasure of intercourse. If, on the other hand, specific sex talk during intimacy is not for you, then say nothing.

One of the biggest sexual turn-offs for a man is when a woman lets herself deteriorate physically. The woman who overeats and then complains about excessive weight is definitely not attractive to the average male. If you have become obese then it is up to you to discipline your eating and take more exercise. I shall be sharing some dieting secrets with you in this book.

Another disclosure made to me by some men concerns female hygiene. The average male who is faced with this problem is reluctant to tell his partner that she is unclean. Of particular concern is the female who has an unpleasant vaginal odour. How can her partner be expected to perform oral sex on her if she smells and tastes awful? Keep in mind how you feel about unhygienic men. Also, check your breath. Who would want to kiss someone with vile breath? With so many toiletries and breath fresheners available today, there really is no excuse for poor personal hygiene.

Another big turn-off for a man is the woman who lives in jeans and big jumpers. Casual wear has its place but not as an unchanging daily uniform. Women should keep in mind that men are more visually aware than females.

Changing the focus from outerwear to underwear, nothing influences a man more than the woman who is dressed in nice lingerie and stockings. A man likes the visual and tactile appeal of stockings which look so feminine and which are silky to the touch. Stockings cover imperfections, add mystery and draw the eye upward – and a man loves that little bit of flesh showing above the stocking tops. Stockings are sexy in a way that tights can never be. Add suspenders to stockings and you have the image of sexual suspense that Hollywood has always been famous for portraying. No Hollywood film has ever portrayed sex by showing a woman in tights.

Today there is such a varied selection of stockings available, including the elasticated top "hold ups", that you are spoilt for choice in style, colour and price range. For something special in hosiery, including fully fashioned stockings, you could see what *What Katie Did* has to offer. Contact details are in the *Appendix*.

Visit any *Erotica* show and you will see that corsets are as popular now as they were in Victorian times, and, no longer are these garments associated with the morally rigid attitude of that period. The temporary demise of the corset was largely due to the fact that corsetry became unfashionable during and after two world wars. Throughout those wars women were doing men's work so corsets became impractical in the work place.

In her shows, Madonna has given the corset a radical new image, consequently bringing this garment back to the forefront as fashionable wear, as did Nicole Kidman in the movie *Moulin Rouge* (2001).

In my work as a sex therapist, I have spoken to a number of call girls on the subject of lingerie. These women tell me that the majority of their male clients insist that they wear corsets and sexy underwear.

Why does the male of the species find corsetry fascinating? I believe one of the reasons that so many men love female foundation wear is because they have past life memories of lives lived in the Victorian era, a time when every woman's body was laced into a corset.

In England we have *Axfords*, a long established (1880) maker of back laced, boned corsets and suspender belts. This Brighton based corsetière is internationally famous for using beautiful materials and producing quality workmanship. To quote from their catalogue, "An *Axfords* corset is made to look and feel beautiful, whether you are wearing it under clothes or as an outer garment. An *Axfords* corset is something special and will make you feel special too."

Axfords garments are stocked through retail outlets as far afield as Japan. You will find contact details for this company in the *Appendix*.

So ladies, do get rid of the shapeless clothing, tights, mismatched lingerie and "baggy" knickers – and transform into a sex goddess. Just remember that the beautiful Venus would never be caught wearing mismatched underwear and knickers that sagged.

In discussing impotence, I have left until last the subject of physical causes, not because the physical aspect is less important but because it is the most obvious. I now deal with some of the health conditions that could cause an erection problem.

A poor diet can adversely affect your sex drive and it is essential that you eat properly for the benefit of your overall health. Check your diet and make sure that you are getting the right balance of food. Having attended to your diet, any of the following five can be taken as a food, such as oats, or a food supplement, as prescribed:

Cardamon (*Elettaria cardamonum*)

Arabs have always regarded this herb as an aphrodisiac which is why some Arab coffee houses mix cardamon with coffee.

Ginger (*Zingiber officinale*)

According to folk medicine, ginger mixed with cardamon will produce an erection.

Gingko (*Gingko biloba*)

This herb improves the flow of blood to the brain. Gingko also boosts the flow of blood to the penis thereby aiding an erection.

Ginseng (*Panax ginseng*: China and Korea)

(*Panax quinquefolium*: North America)

This is another plant that is held in high esteem as an aphrodisiac. Animals are said to increase their sexual activity when they eat ginseng. The Chinese claim that ginseng makes an old man young again.

Horny goat weed (*Epimedium graniflorum*)

This herb is native to China and used in traditional Chinese medicine. A few hundred years ago, a goat herder noticed high levels of sexual activity amongst his goats whenever they ate a certain weed. That weed became known, and still is, as horny goat weed.

Oat (*Avena sativa*)

In the equestrian world stallions become friskier when they are fed oats – so also does the male of the human species, hence the well-known expression "sowing wild oats."

Medical drug dependency, drug abuse, too much alcohol, or excessive smoking, are without a doubt, major contributing causes when dealing with the problem of impotence. Other reasons could be that a man has suffered a pelvic injury, has a heart condition or suffers from diabetes.

Apart from the above mentioned influences, I advise a complete medical check-up to see if there are any hidden problems. If the examination reveals nothing, then I suggest penis pumping. The medical benefits of pumping the penis have been known for many years. A problem in achieving and maintaining an erection is often dispelled by using one of these devices. Ask your doctor for a penis pump or obtain one from an adult sex shop or via the internet.

2

Premature Ejaculation

Premature ejaculation is another worrying problem that more men suffer from than is fully realized. Like impotence, it is a stress situation that generates a high volume of calls to me from men seeking help to deal with this obstacle to a happy sex life.

The men who contact me, most of them nice, normal individuals, do not deny that they call me out of desperation. Most tell me that they have been too embarrassed to ask for medical help, or if they have, they have found their doctors to be unsympathetic.

Astrologically speaking, premature ejaculation is not a problem that is associated with any particular birth sign - it can afflict males from any part of the zodiac, but those under certain zodiac signs are more sensitive to the problem than are those of other star signs. Such was the case with my client Don who was a Leo male… and Leo males like to be slow and perfect lovers.

When Don came to see me for a consultation, he told me that he ejaculated within about five seconds of entering his partner's vagina.

He went on to tell me of his "overwhelming shame" and his inability to discuss the problem, least of all with his partner who he loved very much.

Don said, "After I have finished, I just pull myself out and then turn my back on her and pretend to fall asleep. I am now trying to avoid any sexual contact with her. This is very difficult for me."

Don told me that he had read one of my articles on alternative therapies and had plucked up the courage to ring me. I was pleased that he had made the move to call me and book an appointment.

I asked my client how long he had suffered from the condition.

Don replied, "Always. It didn't matter in the past because sexually I was out for what I could get. But now I'm in love with my partner and I'm afraid it's going to break us up."

With premature ejaculation it is not only the man who suffers. The partner suffers more because at least the man has an orgasm but the woman gains no relief.

The worst part of any difficulty for the man is the humiliation. I explained to Don that there were other ways that he could satisfy his woman. But his shame and concern over premature climaxing was so overwhelming that he had built up a barrier. That barrier was making the problem even worse for the relationship.

I asked Don if his partner had ever talked about the problem. Don told me that she had tried to but when she broached the subject he found himself becoming angry and walked away.

Gently I told Don that anger is often a mask for shame and hurt and that he must talk things out calmly with his partner. I told my client that seventy percent of males ejaculate within minutes of entering the vagina so his problem was not at all unusual. I also pointed out that although most men climax within minutes, women in general need at least fifteen minutes before they climax.

Many men first encounter premature ejaculation during their first sexual experience, a reaction which in most cases is caused by anxiety.

Younger men on average tend to reach orgasm faster than the more experienced older man, but this is not always the case.

Most males, over a period of time, learn to control their orgasms. The difficulty though with many men who have not overcome the problem is that they have not learned to recognize the early warning sensation prior to ejaculation. Learning to control body activity can be likened to the way we learned to control our bladder as children. Some of us took longer than others.

There are various exercises that help deal with the problem of premature ejaculation. One of these exercise programmes is the *stop and start* method which I explained to Don and which I shall explain here.

The exercise programme begins at the start of foreplay.

1. Foreplay should begin and continue until the man's penis becomes erect. At this stage he should lie down on his back and let his female partner masturbate him. It is important that whilst this is happening, the man focuses on the sexual sensation that he is experiencing. When sensing that he is going to climax, he must tell his partner to stop. This exercise should be repeated six times.

After completing this stop and start exercise for the sixth time, the man should either give his partner oral sex or stimulate her clitoris with his fingers. This aspect of the ritual is essential because the woman has just spent time pleasuring her man and she will need some sexual relief too.

Before moving to the next stage, do make sure that you are both comfortable with the exercise procedure so far.

2. This second stage follows the same procedure as the first. The female masturbates her man but this time with the addition of lubrication cream applied to the man's penis. The addition of the cream will increase the sexual sensation.

Do not worry at first if premature ejaculation occurs but employ more sense of control over your feelings. It is crucial that you recognize that early warning sign of a climax on the way – even though the cream is adding extra sensitivity while being masturbated.

3. This part of the programme can either be used as the third and final stage – or as a self-contained and complete exercise in its own right. This is the *squeeze method*. During sexual intercourse, if the man senses that he is about to ejaculate prematurely, he or his partner should squeeze the shaft of his penis between a thumb and two fingers. Pressure is applied just below

the head of the penis for about twenty seconds. Then let go and continue with sex. This technique can be used as often as is necessary.

Some men however find that the best remedy is a desensitising cream or spray used on the penis. Also, condoms will reduce the amount of sensitivity felt during sexual intercourse.

Hypnotherapy too can help with this distressing problem and I have successfully helped many men by using this treatment.

3

Male

Hygiene

Whilst the male secreted chemical pheromone can have a sexually stimulating effect on the female, the opposite reaction will prevail if the male has a poor standard of personal hygiene. Women do not get sexually excited by men who have a strong body odour.

It is important that you smell and taste pleasant for your partner. To help you smell and taste pleasant there is a vast range of deodorants on the market that work well, including the range produced by *The Deodorant Stone (UK) Ltd.* This does not mean that you have to drown yourself in aftershave or cologne. Just have your own sweet, clean body scent, which can, if you wish, be complemented by a subtly scented deodorant or by one of the unscented range such as those made by *The Deodorant Stone.*

Many men forget, or never bother, to regularly wash the whole of their bodies. It is especially important to wash your armpits and genitals. Unwashed, smelly bodies are prone to infection, apart from which, no woman with any sensitivity will want to perform oral sex on a man with a bad genital odour. On that particular subject, please take note of the following.

When having a shower or bath, it is essential for an uncircumcised man to pull back his foreskin and thoroughly wash this area together with the top of his penis. This should be done at least once a day.

Equally important for special attention is the anal area. When you use toilet paper, wipe from the front to the back – and wash your anus too.

A common fault with men is that they forget to keep their hands and nails clean. There is no woman on earth who will let a man with dirty fingernails insert his fingers into her vagina. Not only are dirty fingernails repugnant but they can be the cause of serious infection.

Men should also learn to put on fresh underwear in the morning and change their underwear when they come home in the evening. Dirty underwear is extremely unpleasant for a woman.

Smelly feet are another no-no, very unpleasant indeed, so wash your feet and change your socks regularly. In the cause of promoting healthier feet I recommend *Corrymoor Socks* at Corrymoor Farm, Stockland, Devon, who have a wonderful range of bacteria inhibiting mohair socks, added to which, *Corrymoor's* socks are not only beautifully comfortable and reasonably priced for their excellent quality – but tastefully sexy too.

The worst offenders for smelly feet are trainers. Apart from encouraging foot odour, trainers are ugly, unsexy – and they should only be worn on the sports field where they belong.

My final comment here on the subject of feet is, if you have a serious foot odour problem you should consult your doctor or chemist – and sooner rather than later so that you do not pass on a possible infection to someone else.

Last but not least, teeth and breath. Clean your teeth regularly and gargle frequently with a pleasantly flavoured mouthwash.

4
A
Size Secret
for Men

Does size matter? Many women will respond to that question by saying that it does not matter what a man has, only how he uses what he has. The average male, from an early age though, is obsessed with the size of his penis. Even the most intelligent and sophisticated of men, usually for no good reason, can often feel inadequate where size is concerned. Closer to the truth is the fact that men just want to possess something special between their legs.

In this chapter I give my male readers the secret of how they can improve on what nature gave them.

The exercise system which I describe below originated in the Middle East. This daily exercise is an Arabian stretching technique called *jelqing*. It is a tradition which has been handed down from father to son through the generations.

Before starting the exercise, lubricate your penis. Use only good baby oil or a pure vegetable oil, making sure that you do not use a lubricant which could cause irritation or an allergic reaction.

Now, around the base of your penis make an OK sign with your thumb and forefinger. Use this grip to hold your penis tightly. Gently but firmly slide your forefinger and thumb along the shaft, pulling down and out along the complete length. You will soon experience the head of your penis filling with blood. Repeat this exercise with your other hand, using the same OK grip with your forefinger and thumb.

Continue the milking action with alternate hands. If your penis becomes fully erect, stop immediately and wait until you have a semi erect member.

Practise this exercise five days a week for ten minutes a day in the first week, progressing to fifteen minutes in the second week. Build up to twenty minutes a day thereafter. You should notice a big difference, literally, in the size of your penis after two months.

This exercise technique encourages blood to enter the three cavities of the penis which engorge during an erection. The milking action of the exercise will stretch and expand these chambers and encourage tissue to grow, giving you a larger penis and erection.

I end this chapter by repeating the caution that I mentioned above – never perform jelqing on an erect penis. The reason for this is that you risk causing vascular damage if you do so.

5

Magickal Ways to Lose Weight

Many women come to me asking for magickal help to lose weight. I first suggest to these ladies that they join a weight watchers group where they should be given a sensible diet to follow.

I always add a caution about nutrition and that is; get your doctor's approval before going on any controlled food regime. Along with this advice I recommend certain herbs that are known to witches as enchanted foods. When magickally charged, these particular herbs speed up weight loss. I then advise my weight watchers to start an exercise programme such as yoga which is the subject of the next chapter.

Even before starting any diet it is important to make sure that your body is free from any parasites that invade the human intestinal tract and other parts of the body.

More than one billion people worldwide are host to a variety of intestinal worms. Never make the mistake of thinking that this problem is confined only to developing countries. Many people who complain of being overweight and who suffer from hunger pangs could be infected with worms.

Mainstream medicine has a variety of drugs to treat parasites. These remedies are generally effective, although some of the treatments may cause severe side effects.

I am now going to give you details of a variety of herbs, nuts, seeds and spices that can expel unwanted parasites from your body and speed up your weight loss plan. I will also teach you how to magickally charge herbs so that these plants and special foods have more power when you use them.

Expulsion of parasites

Garlic *(allium sativum)*

Garlic is one of the oldest natural remedies for removing intestinal worms. Garlic can be used in various ways such as adding the juice of three garlic cloves to between four and six ounces of carrot juice. This drink should be taken every two hours.

Pumpkin *(Cucurbita pepo)*

Pumpkin seeds have been shown to immobilise and aid in the expulsion of intestinal worms and parasites.

Walnut *(Jugulans regia)*

When you are dieting take a handful of walnuts every day. The nuts not only stop the craving for food but they also expel worms from the intestinal tract.

Weight loss

Chickweed *(Stellaria media)*

Chickweed, which can be found in abundance in Britain, can be used in its fresh state for most of the year. Chickweed is known for its laxative property.

Dandelion *(Taraxacum officinale)*

Dandelion leaves and the juice of the dandelion plant's root are useful in any diet. Both can help to purify the blood and reduce water retention in the body.

Hot spices

In a research project scientists measured the metabolic rate of their volunteers' standard diet. A teaspoon of red pepper sauce and a teaspoon of mustard were then added to every subject's meal. The hot condiments raised the research volunteers' metabolic rates by as much as twenty-five percent.

Hot spices stimulate thirst so you drink more and eat less and, by doing so, you take in fewer calories.

Walnut *(Juglans regia)*

The walnut is mentioned again here as a reminder that walnuts are not only good for expelling worms but, relevant to weight loss, cut down on the craving for food; providing a natural and tasty treat for your weight watchers programme.

Magickally charging herbs

Just imagine that you have decided to use some dandelion leaves as part of your dieting project. To charge the leaves - or any plants, just put the amount that you need in a bowl. Then put your hands over the bowl and close your eyes. Now feel the energy rising from the dandelion leaves. Touch the leaves with your dominant hand while your eyes are still closed. Then concentrate on your magickal need – in this case ridding yourself of internal parasites. Now hold some of the leaves in your hand and rub them between your fingers. Feel the exchange of energy flowing between you and the dandelion leaves. You now have the secret of charging your plants for a magickal purpose.

Now some words of caution. When gathering herbs in the countryside, do make sure that you collect your plants in an area free from chemical spraying, discarded rubbish – and places where people walk dogs.

When you get home, thoroughly wash and rinse the herbs before consumption.

To conclude, let me advise you that Tuesday is a very good day to start your weight loss programme. Tuesday is ruled by Mars symbolizing the masculine energy involved in conflict, physical endurance and strength. Any failed weight watcher will know about conflict and physical endurance when trying to keep to a diet.

6

Once
the Secret
of the Yogis

A lack of exercise is obviously one of the major causes of bulging bodies. For many of us though, the thought of jogging, or nearly killing ourselves in a gymnasium, is a nightmare.

The answer to a balanced exercise routine has to be … YOGA. This centuries old system of postures is gentle and civilised; there are no side effects, and believe it or not, you do not have to stand on your head to benefit.

The beauty of yoga is that you can learn the exercises by attending classes or just teach yourself the system from a book. You can then practise the postures anywhere – at home, in a desert, on top of a mountain – or in the middle of a forest.

Hatha yoga is the most common form of yoga practised in the West but kundalini yoga came to the forefront in 2000 when *The Eight Human Talents* by Gurmukh was published. Gurmukh attracted students such as Madonna, David Duchovny, Cindy Crawford, Rosanna Arquette and Flea of the *Red Hot Chili Peppers,* all of whom praised Gurmukh for the way in which Kundalini yoga had helped them.

Yoga provides exercise postures that address such ailments as asthma, addiction, anaemia, insomnia, stress, senility, our old enemy obesity, and a multitude of other health conditions. Not only does yoga deal with numerous problems that are present, but the exercises boost the immune system for the future.

Yoga is a mind-body-spirit therapy, but if you are only looking for physical benefit, the system will give you just that. If you are looking for mental and spiritual balance, the system will give you that too. Yoga, on any or all three levels, can take you from what you have become to what you want to be – and what you should be. And, as I have emphasized in the *Erection Problems* chapter, you need all aspects of yourself in balance to have a fulfilling sex life.

After practising yoga every day for only two weeks you should notice that changes have taken place. You will have more energy, a more positive mental attitude and more interest in life. The changes may be subtle but the changes will be there. Continue practising these mystical exercises and you should be on a permanent path to the proper weight, overall good physical and mental health – and a more satisfying sex life.

And a word or two for the men; there is no need to react to yoga in the way that you might if someone suggested that you take up knitting or flower arranging. Remember that these exercises originated from the wise men of India.

7

Sex Fantasies

Many of my clients worry about having sexual fantasies that do not include their partners. They feel guilty about committing a kind of fantasy infidelity.

Interestingly, research has shown that those who fantasize the most are likely to be in the happiest of relationships.

If you are one of the unfortunate few who cannot talk about your fantasies with your partner, then an imaginary scenario presents you with a free hand to play out any sexual role or scene that you wish. You can be truly creative and write your own script.

If you find it difficult to fantasize about sex, you can always use illustrated sex magazines and adult movies as a trigger for a fantasy. Just visit your local licensed sex shop, have a look at what is on offer - and choose accordingly.

Here are some of the common male fantasies:

- ♦ Having sex with a partner who is wearing sexy underwear
- ♦ Giving and receiving oral sex
- ♦ Three in a bed
- ♦ Watching others having sex

Here are some of the common female fantasies:

- ♦ Having sex with her partner
- ♦ Having sex with a new partner
- ♦ Being submissive
- ♦ Indulging in forbidden sex

Some couples find it wonderful to share and act out their fantasies together while one or the other of a conventional couple would not be happy to do so.

Each person's fantasy is very personal, particularly if the imaginary scenario involves an aspect of the individual's sexuality that is normally hidden from view.

My advice, if you are uncertain about your partner's view on fantasies, is to talk about the general theme of your imaginary sex games and then gauge the reaction. Be cautious though.

8
Pleasuring
Your Sexual Self

Single people often tell me that they feel guilty about self-pleasuring. Here we have yet another area of sexual activity that can often cause a feeling of shame. It is sad that such a magickal activity as sex, often, for the wrong reasons, triggers feelings of guilt which may turn into neurosis and even psychosis.

Let me start off here by saying that... **masturbation is perfectly normal**.

There will always be some "moral" busybody somewhere, either in the shape of an individual or of some organization, who will view masturbation as the sign of a downward spiral into degeneracy. "Playing with yourself" has been promoted, for example, by the Church at one time or another as an activity that will guarantee you a place in purgatory.

Thank goodness that today people are more cynical about being lectured, particularly after the all too numerous scandals involving members of the supposed moral guardians of our society. Nevertheless, there are still many decent people who feel guilty about sex and their sexuality. If this were not so, my counselling would not be needed by so many.

Let me repeat that self-pleasuring is quite normal. If you allow yourself to go with the flow of your sexual feelings, masturbation can be very pleasurable. I shall now give you some tips so that you can make masturbation even more pleasing.

Self-pleasuring can be all the more satisfying if you vary the ways in which you touch yourself. Self-exploration is the key factor because no-one is born with the knowledge of how their body responds to various kinds of stimulation. It is a matter of learning which part of you responds to what. We are all different and the only way to find out what pleases us is by experimenting.

Try stimulating those areas of your body that particularly excite you but avoid the obvious - such as the clitoris and the penis. If you stimulate your clitoris or penis you will probably climax too quickly and lose the joy of finding other satisfying arousal places - so explore other areas of your body first.

Try an application of oil or cream when you touch yourself. See how you react to the sensation of a soft body brush. Perhaps you will like the sensual feel of a silk scarf next to the skin - or a feather as I suggested in *The Sex Magick Feather Massage*.

If you have a spouse or partner then you can "sex-up" your sex life with mutual masturbation. There are several advantages to mutual masturbation. There is no risk of infection; there is no risk of pregnancy; it is not physically harmful – and for the male with an erection problem there is no pressure to "perform".

You can also ask your partner to masturbate while you watch. Apart from the voyeuristic appeal, there is much to be learned from watching someone self-pleasure.

The Goddess has given us the magickal orgasm so I wish you well in finding new ways to achieve that special moment of ecstasy.

9

Senior Sex Anyone?

There are still some who feel that when men and women retire, their respective sex organs should be retired too. Some typical sentiments expressed by those who hold such a view are, "The thought of oldies 'doing it' is not very nice," or, "He's a 'dirty old man'".

At a time when "grey power" people have become a fashionable media subject, there is often a space left where there could be a sensible and sensitive discussion about whether those of a certain age have power in their sex lives too. The general image of the over sixties is that they are the *over sexties* – not oversexed but over sex. Nothing could be further from the truth for many senior citizens. Sadly though, some fall into the trap of thinking that the only activity left to them is putting on their carpet slippers.

For those of you who are post menopause – and I include men in this category, now is a very good time to have some fun because, apart from anything else, you can concentrate on your sexual pleasure without the worry of an unwanted pregnancy.

You may no longer be able to dance the Charleston or swing from a chandelier but you can still enjoy the sensual and erotic pleasure of an intimate touch – and much more besides - unless you have a serious health condition that prevents sexual activity.

So, particularly relevant is the importance of keeping fit, because the fitter you are, the better your sex will be.

Watching your diet and taking regular exercise such as walking, cycling, swimming and gardening, will improve your muscle tone and help you to maintain a healthy cardiac system. For those who practise yoga, do continue with this amazingly beneficial system of exercises.

The overall benefit of exercising regularly is that you will age less quickly together with the added bonus of enjoying good sex. And, an active sex life produces a variety of chemicals that will help you to keep happy, improve your immune system and thicken skin tissue. By improving and continuing with your sex lives you can look up to seven years younger than you are.

When we pass a certain age, most of the physical changes that take place are due to the natural aging process. This is evident when skin loses its sensitivity and body movement becomes restricted. Both men and women will experience hormonal changes as they go through the transformation of the menopause.

After the menopause many women complain that they have less sexual desire. Men also complain that their desire for sex is less frequent and less urgent than when they were in their twenties.

Women generally find that it takes them longer to reach a climax and that the sensation of their orgasm is weaker. Men find that they have a longer arousal time and that they need direct penis stimulation to get an erection. And, although men can achieve penetration of the vagina, they find that their erection is not as hard as it was. But, one of the joys of grey sex is that men take longer to reach their climax, so not only will they enjoy sex more but so too will their partners.

It is important to be aware of your bodily changes as you go through the age transition. You can then make the necessary adjustments to your love-making. Sex changes with age but that does not mean that your love life has to be less enjoyable.

As a sex witch, I know there are many senior citizens who are sexually active, and, unlike those delightful characters in the *Cocoon* movies, the folk I am thinking of have never had the benefit of extra terrestrials to help them with their love lives.

I have so often noticed that these active "oldies" are really happy people with a glow and a twinkle in their eyes – and that speaks volumes.

Whatever your age, I wish you a happy and fulfilling sex life.

10

Geopathic Stress – The Unseen Force

This is the force that you do **not** want to be with you. I am talking about the underground and ground level negative energy areas that are often referred to as geopathically stressed.

There are known minerals and rocks, granite is an example of the latter, which hold and release a radioactive gas known as radon. This gas can have a lethal effect on your health.

Overhead power lines too, some of which carry 400,000 volts, also disturb nature's natural balance and harmony – and your balance and harmony as well. Additional problems are roads (particularly motorways), railways, underground mines and quarries. These man-made structures and earth disturbances are either cutting across or digging into or under the ground's surface. Such wounding seriously disturbs our planet's energy field and that disturbance can be passed on to you – if you are too close to such a stress imbalance.

The subject of geopathic stress highlights the story of Helen and her partner who had done nothing but argue since moving into their new home. In fact, the situation had deteriorated to the point where they rarely made love. Helen was very worried and wondered if the house had been cursed.

When Helen came to see me, I asked if, apart from a lack of sexual activity, there were any other physical problems. She told me that her partner was taking medication for depression and that she had not had a good night's sleep since moving into their new home.

I asked Helen how her home felt and she told me that the atmosphere was not very friendly or "good".

All the signs pointed to the house being geopathically stressed, a common factor in many major as well as minor illnesses.

Here are just some of the many health problems that can be linked to GS: infertility, miscarriages, lack of libido, exhaustion, depression, food allergies and also cancer. Geopathic stress therefore is something that you do not want to encounter too closely for too long.

The advice that I gave Helen is the same guidance that I will give you further down when dealing with negative energy.

The ancients knew all about the Earth's energies and they were aware of areas that they had to be careful of. Our ancient ancestors would leave cattle on intended building land for one year to test the ground. The cattle were then slaughtered and their entrails inspected for signs of abnormality. On the basis of what was found, a decision was made as to whether to build or not to build on the land in question.

Gypsies, who move from place to place, seldom suffer from chronic illnesses and generally enjoy good health. This is interesting because many of them smoke and drink, use salt and sugar freely in their food and never bother about a special diet. But gypsies do bother about where they settle for any given period of time. They know about negative forces in the ground and avoid such areas at all cost.

These facts were recorded in a survey carried out by Christopher McNaney of the People's Research Centre, Alston, and are mentioned in Rolf Gordon's book *Are You Sleeping in a Safe Place?* But many witches who mix with, or who are familiar with the Romany lifestyle, also know this to be true. Gypsies break all the accepted rules of healthy living and get away with it because they know something the majority of the population are completely unaware of. Gypsies know about geopathic stress.

Animals are more psychic than humans and tune into the Earth's radiation. Just look where your pet cat or dog chooses to settle in the house or in the garden. Take note too of the areas that your pet avoids. Also ask yourself if you feel less comfortable in some parts of your home than you do in other areas. These are simple ways of checking for negative energy. You could also try to find out if the previous occupants of your home suffered from a series of health problems, whether the woman of the house had a miscarriage or if there was a divorce. These unfortunate situations are often pointers to the possibility that a building is geopathically stressed.

If you do suspect that there is GS affecting your home I advise you to call in a dowser or feng shui consultant who will be able to pinpoint any area of negative energy. The *British Society of Dowsers* at Malvern, Worcestershire, should be able to give you the name of your local dowser.

If you like doing your own dowsing, the *Centre for Implosion Research* at Bristol have for sale dowsing rods for detection and also various purpose-made devices that help protect against geopathic stress and electromagnetic pollution.

The *Centre's* contact details are given in the *Appendix*. Also listed at the back of this book is *Dulwich Health* whose director Rolf Gordon has authored *Are You Sleeping in a Safe Place?* This detailed manual, now in its seventh edition, is packed with information about GS including detailed guidance on how to search for and deal with negative energy. There are over eighty different subject headings in the book which include the sad story of the death of Rolf Gordon's son from testicular cancer. This tragedy put the author on the path of investigating and publicizing the lethal effects of geopathic stress.

You can also add to your reading list *Geopathic Stress – how Earth energies affect our lives* by Jane Thurnell-Read. These two books should tell you everything you need to know about GS.

Here are some measures that you can take to help eliminate negative energy. Magnets can correct some disturbances caused by negative energy. Place magnets on incoming water pipes and electric cables – and please take care with the latter.

A magickal way of dealing with geopathic stress is to take a photograph of your home and bury the picture in your back garden. Also have indoor plants such as Boston ferns around the house because plants help to remove environmental pollutants. Quartz crystals placed near television sets and computers add to your protection too. Last but not least, as I mention in the *Sex Magick* chapter, if you have exposed overhead beams, suspend some wind chimes or crystals from these supports because exposed ceiling beams are bad for relationships.

Another source of unseen negative energy can often be a resident earthbound spirit. In many cases these souls have died under unfortunate circumstances such as suicide or murder.

Homes and buildings that are haunted by an unhappy spirit often have an oppressive, dank and dark broodiness that no amount of light will clear. One of the other clues that can indicate a spirit presence in a house is if the building has a distinctive cold spot somewhere. The spirit presence and the attendant atmosphere that it has created can overshadow all who live in the house, causing depression and sickness.

If you suspect that you have an unhappy spirit in your home, call in a psychic or medium for a consultation. One of the team at the *Two World's* journal should be able to give you the name of a medium in your area if you need help.

Perhaps you have a resident spirit who is not a real problem but you would feel just a little bit happier without its presence. If that is the case then you can try the DIY advice that I give in the chapter *The Home That Became a Haunted "House"*.

May the force be with you, the positive force that is, not the negative.

11

The Responsible Use of Herbs

Herbs can cure – or kill. In this book you will find a variety of herbs recommended so I start this chapter with the above caution.

The ingredients and chemical compounds that are present in herbs and plants are numerous and varied in their strengths to cure, induce altered states of consciousness – or kill. In the latter case, belladonna, also known as deadly nightshade *(Atropa Belladonna)**, hemlock *(Conium maculatum)*, and henbane *(Hyoscyamus niger)*, are three well-known killers.

You will not find belladonna, hemlock or henbane on my recommended list. Nor will you find the delicate petalled opium poppy *(Papaver somniferum)*, whose unripe seed pod milk induces a deep, altered state of consciousness.

You will though, find that the herbs mentioned in this book are recommended for their benefits in the context of the subject under discussion – and for their remedial properties.

If you decide to try one or more of the herbal remedies that I recommend in *A WITCH'S GUIDE,* you should first seek dosage guidance from a registered herbalist or your local complementary health centre or shop.

Some of the nightshade family contain the poisonous alkaloid scopolamine, a clear liquid substance that was used as a truth drug by the *Geheime Staatspolizei (Gestapo)*, in Nazi Germany.

You will also need special guidance with regard to herbal remedies if you are taking medication or suffer from an allergy. Then there are certain herbs which should not be taken by pregnant women.

The best herbs that you can use, whether for medicinal or culinary purposes, are those that are fresh – and there are none fresher than those that you grow yourself.

It is very easy to create your own herb garden or grow your own plants in pots if you lack garden space. It will not take long before you have your own stock of magickal and medicinal herbs.

Alternatively, if you buy herbs from a commercial supplier, do make sure that the plants have been organically grown. Often the best way to find a reliable organic source of supply is through word of mouth recommendation.

Good luck with your herb garden. Plant cultivation is a truly magickal pastime and the more things we grow, whatever they may be, the more we help our environment and Mother Earth.

Some final cautions; never pick and sample any herb or a part of any herb that you are unable to identify, even if the plant looks familiar. Only pick and use herbs that you can positively identify – and collected away from areas frequented by dog walkers or from motorways where plants will be contaminated by vehicle fumes.

Section 5
Sexual Characteristics Revealed

1
The Sexual Aura

Every one of us is surrounded by an electromagnetic energy field which is expressed in a combination of colours. This energy field, called the aura, indicates our physical and spiritual state at any given time. The colours in the aura also reveal our sexual orientation and experiences from our past, present and, incredibly our future incarnations.

In alphabetical order below are the colours and shades of the aura that reveal our sexual make-up, starting with black, which is the most negative of the aura's colour spectrum.

Black
It is rare to find black in someone's aura. However, when black does appear, it indicates a totally negative and obsessive personality. Someone with such an aura is usually involved in the stranger side of sexual activities. This type tends to be cruel and could commit a sexually motivated murder.

A good example of a black personality would be the serial killer known as Jack the Ripper. In the late nineteenth century Jack brutally killed several prostitutes in the East End of London.

Another example would be Charles Manson who, with his "family", murdered nine people in California in 1969. One of their victims was Hollywood actress Sharon Tate who at the time was married to film director Roman Polanski the director of the satanic themed movie *Rosemary's Baby* (1968). In that film with a small acting part was the late leader of the *Church of Satan* Anton LaVey. Fact is indeed stranger than fiction.

Blue

Someone with blue in their aura will be good at "sweet talking". Although likely to be insincere, this individual, even if physically unattractive, will impress as an absolute charmer. A blue person is excellent at making someone feel very special.

Gold

Gold in the aura is an expression of spirituality and a love of people.

A gold person is very particular, fussy with detail, and always puts a high value on cleanliness. A gold person also has impeccable taste and likes designer clothes.

Many gay people who typically have these characteristics have gold in their auras.

Green

Someone with a lot of green in his or her energy field is normally faithful. Such a person will also have an understanding and forgiving nature.

A dark green personality however, can be jealous and envious. This is the type who will also marry for material gain. A dark green person can dispense with genuine love and would not think twice about making love to someone in order to raise their own status in life. Both female and male opportunists will have dark green in their auras.

Orange

Orange in the aura is an expression of a sporty, party-loving personality. Such an individual is good natured and generous.

An abundance of orange in the aura is often the characteristic of swingers who enjoy sex with a lot of different partners. A woman with a large amount of orange in her energy field is usually bisexual or she has bisexual tendencies.

On the negative side, overindulging in sex can backfire and create emotional problems for an orange person.

Red

Someone with a generous amount of red in their aura will have an energetic and uninhibited sexual appetite. A working girl (prostitute) will have a lot of red in her pelvic region.

On the negative side, I have seen adults and children with red in their pelvic area which is a sure sign that they have suffered some kind of sexual abuse. If a light shade of red is shown, this usually indicates that the abuse has been inflicted in a past incarnation. However, if the shade seen is between a deep and a burgundy red, then abuse is taking place in that person's present life.

Violet

A violet person will appreciate Tantric sex and sex magick. Such a person will be good at massage and will take time to please a lover. Foreplay is important to a violet person who will often use sex toys.

Someone with a deeper, purple toned colour in his or her aura could make a good living at writing sex novels or talking on telephone sex lines. A purple person likes to talk in explicit sexual terms. Purple people are also frequently pornographic movie directors.

Yellow

Light yellow in the aura indicates a self-controlled, confident person. A deeper yellow expresses an egotistical personality who likes to control.

A dark yellow person fears losing respect and will need to be in charge. Such a personality is drawn to sadism and bondage and will enjoy administering punishment. This type will make an ideal partner for someone who is submissive.

White

Bright white in an aura is unusual. When bright white does occur in the energy field, it usually belongs to someone who is not particularly interested in sex.

A dull white indicates a fear of sex. Such a person will suffer from depression and keep apart from others. This type of personality is the typical loner. A pale white around the hips indicates a person who died a virgin in a previous life.

Note: The human aura can be photographed by a process known as *Kirlian* photography. See the *Information Section* for details.

2

Handwriting Secrets

People do not realize when they are writing that the way they dot their i's and cross their t's will say more about them than they may realize. We do not have to think too hard before we transform our thoughts to paper. We express those thoughts, and our feelings, through the automatic action of handwriting, a social custom for communicating with one another. Handwriting is such a routine habit that we are unaware that our writing style reveals who we really are to the trained eye.

As we get older, health and personality traits show more clearly in the way we write. Our handwriting therefore becomes as distinctive as a fingerprint or DNA pattern.

Here are some telltale signs to look for when analyzing handwriting:

Should you want to know if your partner is a pathological liar, just look at the way he forms his Os. This vowel is a letter of communication which, according to the way it is written, can indicate secretiveness, sexual affairs, self deceit, indiscreet talk and frankness.

The pathological liar will form his Os with two huge inner loops in both halves of this vowel, so beware if your partner writes his Os in this fashion.

A domineering personality who likes to control can be identified by the handwriting characteristic of a right slanting t bar. A dominatrix more often than not will have this particular t bar giveaway in her writing.

A low t bar indicates low self-esteem. Sexually submissive people often cross their t's with low t bars.

It is easy to identify someone's sexual make-up by the way the person writes loops on lower case letters. For example, long and wide loops on the y or g will belong to a wonderful lover. However, this type will easily become bored, so experiment with your lovemaking to hold such a person's interest.

People who write with long and wide loops are often to be found in swinging and gay communities.

If you are looking for a partner who likes responsibility, then look for someone who forms large loops at the beginning of capital letters, usually W or M. Large looped males, so to speak, will never forget to wear a condom.

Handwriting which is wild distinguishes a creative personality, and most likely indicates someone who is good at erotic writing. The German composer Ludwig van Beethoven possessed such a style of lettering.

With the examples that I have given in this chapter I have demonstrated that the way you write is the way you are, and the study of handwriting, called graphology, is a fascinating hobby and a lifetime study for the graphologist.

3

More Secrets at Hand

Throughout my working life I have examined the hands of murderers, thieves, cheats, liars, those with unusual sexual preferences and yes, the hands of some nice, honest, sensitive and charming people too.

Hand **lines**, like hand **writing**, reveal much more than some of us would wish to have revealed. Our hands present the trained eye with a picture of who we really are. However, many palmists may not be able to decipher a subject's sexual characteristics.

As a sex witch I have studied palmistry with an emphasis on sexual character analysis. The hand provides me with a detailed diagram of a subject's sexual traits - characteristics that are in a code language of lines, mounts and the shape of the hand and fingers.

Human hands are truly amazing. Each hand has twenty-seven bones, dozens of muscles and millions of nerves.

We perform a thousand and one tasks with our hands which can also be our physical expression of tenderness, sensitivity and love – or they can be the tools of aggression with which to hit, maim and kill.

Hands and fingers come in all shapes and sizes and these individual differences give the palmist and psychic their first indication of a subject's personality.

For example, someone with spatulate hands will be active, energetic, self-confident and will tend to be very practical and grounded.

The sexual profile of this particular subject will be of one who often indulges in quick sex and has a liking for pornography.

Another category of personality is the individual with psychic hands

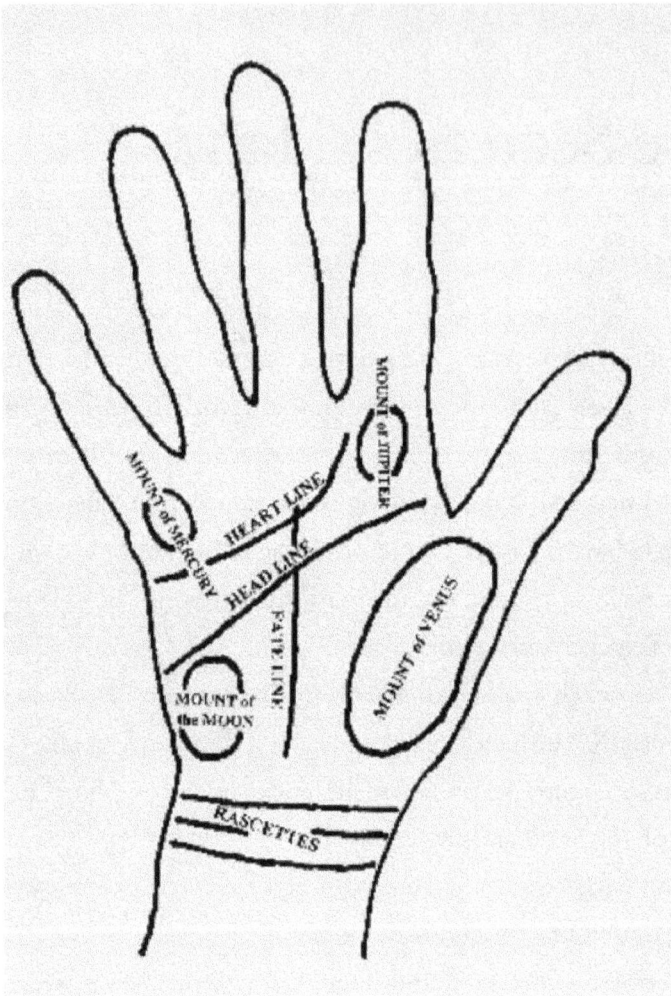

which are quite distinctive and not very common. The fingers of such a hand are long and pointed and belong to one who is sensitive. This person will like sex fantasy enactment and will often act out a role with a willing partner. Many who have psychic hands are gay or bisexual.

The human hand has etched upon it an amazingly complex network of lines - but there are only three major lines; the lines of head, heart and fate. All three should be seen clearly etched on the palm.

I have deliberately omitted the life line because this line can be inaccurate in predicting a subject's life span. I have from time to time seen a long life line on a palm but known that the person in front of me has only a short time to live. The fate line will give me a far more accurate indication of longevity.

Head line

The head line indicates our mental capacity, intellectual skill and sexual make-up.

A subject with a noticeably long, strong and straight head line will be sexually experienced and confident.

A weak head line could indicate a nervous breakdown or a series of breakdowns.

Beware of one who has a head line which goes without any curve in a straight line across the palm. This characteristic belongs to an individual who is drawn to someone's material worth rather than their sexuality.

Watch out too for the person with a wavy head line. This type is usually a confidence trickster who should not be trusted - either in love or business.

If your partner has a head line that splits at the end with one of the splits dropping down toward the top of the wrist and the other split going up to touch the heart line, you have someone who will give up all for love.

A short head line usually belongs to an unhappy person who is likely to be prone to accidents and sudden illnesses.

A garland type of configuration under the head line usually means that the person concerned suffers from migraine attacks and often has a fear of sex. Regular masturbation or sexual intercourse will often cure this condition.

Heart line

The heart line records affairs of the heart. When you interpret this particular line, you have an insight and numerous clues to the subject's sexual temperament and compatibility regarding relationships.

If for example, a couple possess fragmented heart lines, indicating emotional temperaments, then they may experience a problem in their relationship. However, their time together will never be boring.

A long straight heart line running across a person's palm will almost always indicate emotional coldness. This person's partner will never feel secure and could be in a relationship with someone possessing sadistic tendencies.

Fate line

The fate line is located in the middle of the palm, usually running vertically from the base of the palm, just above the wrist, and heading toward the third finger. This line has very important significance for career/work opportunities. When the fate line runs its full length in a clean, strong, unbroken trace, such a feature indicates that the subject will have a secure career – and a good sex life.

Let me point out here that a weak fate line is not an indication of a short life. Many of my clients have expressed concern about possessing a weak fate line. Such a characteristic does not signal a short life. However, if the line is short, fades out or becomes wispy, this does suggest delicate health or the loss of a will to live.

This type of individual often has a take it or leave it attitude to sex, but, if motivated, can make an excellent lover.

I shall now move on to analyzing the mounts on the palm of the hand. These fleshy pads can be interpreted to add more revealing insights about the sexual personality.

Mount of the Moon

The Moon mount starts by the wrist and goes half way up the palm toward the little finger. This palm pad expresses our loving and sexual nature.

A medium size Moon mount reveals an imaginative person. This individual will be a very romantic and skilled lover.

A high Moon mount will be possessed by someone who is more

interested in the mystic arts than in sex. Tantric sex may be the answer for this type.

An over large Moon mount will belong to a person who is economical with the truth. Such a subject will have difficulty in separating truth from fantasy.

Someone with a flat Moon mount will lack imagination – a trait that will be taken into the bedroom for some boring sex.

Mount of Jupiter

The Jupiter mount is located at the top of the palm beneath the base of the index finger.

A Jupiter mount of medium thickness expresses a self-confident, generous person who commands respect. Such an individual is fantastic in bed and will do anything to please.

A high Jupiter mount belongs to someone who likes a peaceful life. This subject can be tedious in bed and will tend not to vary from the same lovemaking position.

Watch out for the individual who has an abnormally large Jupiter mount. This type is arrogant, overbearing and can be a bully.

The gold digger who marries for gain rather than love also has a very large Jupiter mount.

A flat Jupiter mount belongs to a lazy, selfish individual who is selfish in bed too. It will be he who reaches his climax first before thoughtlessly rolling away and going to sleep.

Mount of Mercury

The Mercury mount is located at the top of the palm beneath the fourth finger.

A subject with a medium Mercury mount will be good at mathematics.

Apart from mathematics, what distinguishes this individual is an urge to go where others fear to tread. Possessed with charm, this subject likes an adventurous sex life and will often be drawn to bondage.

A high Mercury mount reveals someone with a good sense of humour - but one who should be made to realize that there is a person behind the gags. This joker will laugh you into bed.

Mount of Venus

The mount of Venus is located below the base of the thumb, forming a ball that is half encircled by the life line.

The Venus mount reveals our ability to let go of inhibitions, our love of love and sex, our attraction to the luxurious things in life – and our sensitivity.

A medium Venus mount reveals a warm, magnetic person. This subject has vitality and stamina and will be a virile lover.

A high Venus mount is possessed by someone who will lead a sleazy life-style and overindulge in everything from food and drink to sex.

A flat Venus mount is the sign of someone with a low sex drive. Such individuals are usually cold and unaffectionate.

Rascettes and other hand language coding

A rascette or bracelet, which appears at the wrist, is seen as indicating thirty years of life. Three distinct rascettes therefore indicate ninety years of life.

Let me say that this measurement is only a guideline. Nevertheless, clear bracelets do indicate strength, a good immune system and longevity. Clear rascettes also point to sexual stamina.

Hand colour

Healthy hands should have a good natural colour appropriate to the race or ethnic group to which they belong.

Hands should be firm to the touch, and, bearing in mind prevailing weather conditions, should be pleasantly warm.

Brown

Brown patches, apart from age spots, could suggest tumours or a blockage somewhere.

Psychologically, brown patch people tend to hang on to past hurts without letting go. An insult, particularly about their sexual performance, would stay with them forever.

Blue-grey or mauve

Someone with blue-grey or mauve colouration around the fingers could have poor circulation and even a weak heart. Blue-grey people are often emotionally closed down and can only show love through sex.

Red

Red hands indicate thyroid or blood pressure problems.

A red hand person, rather than enjoying sex, will worry about his or her sexual performance.

White

White hands may be an expression of anaemia and, as with blue-greys, also poor circulation. These folk often feel too tired for sex.

Yellow

Yellow hands suggest a liver problem. Not surprisingly, such hands often belong to an alcoholic. With that in mind, there is little that one can say about such an individual's sex life.

Other hand conditions

Whether hot, cold, clammy or soft, each of these hand conditions tells a story.

Clammy hands

Clammy hands are the expression of a sluggish liver. Someone with this sticky characteristic will have a tendency to cling to past anger and arguments. In some cases a clammy hand person can be violent. Keep this in mind where a relationship is concerned.

Cold hands

Cold, dry hands may indicate circulation problems or the onset of an illness.

A man with cold hands could suffer from impotence.

Hot, dry hands

Hot, dry hands often express a blood pressure problem, a kidney complication or simply the beginning of a feverish infection. A person in this category may often carry a sexual secret from childhood.

Hot, sweaty hands

Hot, sweaty hands may be due to a thyroid problem or some other glandular complication.

You are probably thinking that I am stating the obvious when I say that peeping Toms and flashers have sweaty hands too. Well, I am just confirming your suspicions.

Soft hands

It is perfectly normal for elderly people to have soft hands. The same applies to pregnant women and vegetarians, apart from which, this characteristic could be a sign of weak health.

Psychologically, soft hands can indicate a passive nature. In a sexual context, soft hands often point to a masochist or someone who enjoys playing a sex slave role.

So there you are; hands lines and hands provide the palmist and the psychic with an incredible amount of information about the subject's sexual persona and individual personality.

Hand Analyses

Hand 1 Female

I see this person as one who was liberated before feminism became fashionable. She is a traditionalist who values good manners - and a romantic who appreciates roses and chocolates from the man in her life. This subject is artistic, self critical, a perfectionist and a genuine humanitarian who enjoys helping others. She is in charge of her own destiny and also mistress of her own sex life.

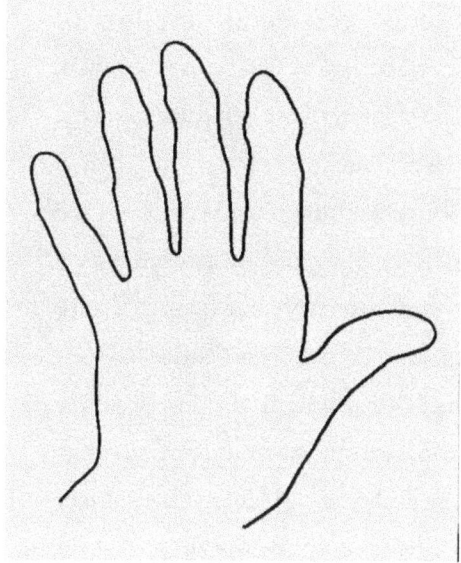

Hand 2 Male

This subject was aware of his individual sexuality from an early age. He is psychic, diplomatic and a good communicator. He is also thorough and would make a good investigative journalist. He has a genuine objective interest in sex and does not judge the sexual orientations of others. It is important that he expresses himself sexually otherwise depression sets in. This characteristic was stronger in his early years.

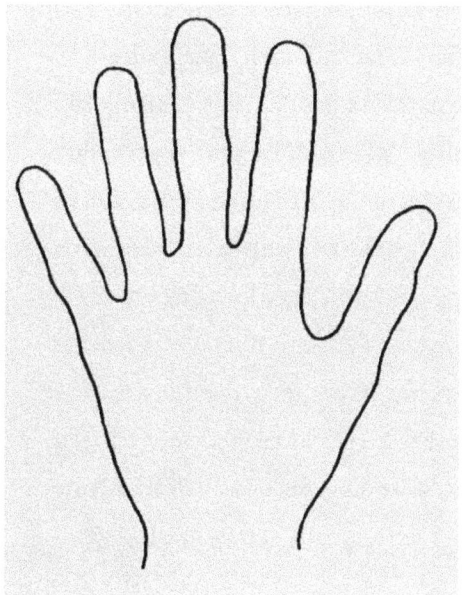

Hand 3 Female

She arouses the protective instinct in men but resents any loss of independence. With this individual, social intercourse can turn to sexual intercourse, for a good conversationalist turns her on. I see her, in her past or present, as a songwriter with star quality. There is also a practical side to this individual which she applies in a professional capacity. She also has the ability to sell ideas. This subject enjoys good, healthy sex.

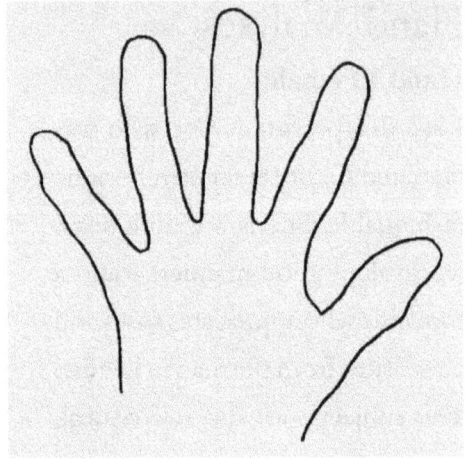

Hand 4 Male

I see this subject as a gay male who likes beautiful men. Size matters to this individual. He has a strong sex drive with a dominant personality to match. Unfortunately, he adopts an authoritarian attitude with people and has lost friends as a result. Although not an actor, actor would have been the ideal career for this individual who sees himself as a leading man modeled on one of yesteryear's screen idols.

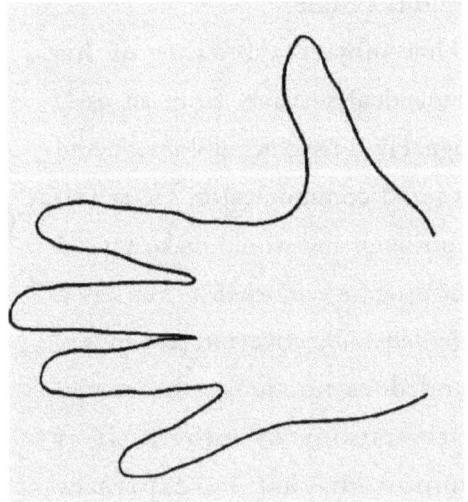

You will see from the hand silhouettes that there are distinctive differences between finger and palm shapes and sizes. From these patterns I have used my own method of deduction to arrive at the four character readings given here. I have never met any of the four subjects although I do know one through telephone conversations and correspondence. The four hand outlines were contributed upon the understanding of anonymity. The only other information given was specific birth dates for each individual. These dates are omitted here to respect the privacy of the contributors.

4

Your Birth Sign is Your Sex Sign

At the time we incarnate we acquire the influence of the birth sign under which we are born, giving us a particular kind of personality imprint.

A significant and obviously important part of that personality imprint is the sexual aspect. Revealed here are the sexual identities not only of your birth sign but of the other eleven signs too.

ARIES March 21ˢᵗ to April 20ᵗʰ

Aries is the first sign of the zodiac and a fire sign – an appropriate element for Ariens because they like to live dangerously and play with fire where sex is concerned.

Having sex in strange places with the risk of getting caught for example, adds a certain edge.

Another turn-on for daring Ariens is that they like their sex in front of appreciative strangers. When this sexual exhibitionism takes place outdoors it is known as dogging.

The Aries woman loves oral sex – and she likes to give as well as to receive such intimate stimulation.

The Aries man likes quickies. For an outstanding sexual effect he favours black condoms.

A negative aspect of Ariens is that they can be rough and selfish with their love-making.

TAURUS April 21st to May 21st

Taurus is an earth sign.

Taureans are very sensual people who love sex but do not indulge in anything outrageous.

Good food and conversation can be as important as good sex to Taureans. Being "foodies", they appreciate any kind of love food and will choose fruit or chocolate flavoured condoms to please a partner – along with chocolate body paint.

Some Taurean males suffer from sexual hang-ups and there are Taurean women who have no significant sexual experiences until late in life.

GEMINI May 22nd to June 21st

Gemini's element is air. It is one of the intellectual signs of the zodiac.

Geminis are easily bored so they will search for fresh sexual stimulation and be willing to try anything once.

Their search for new sex games will often lead them into threesome scenarios.

Many Geminis are bisexual but they will not admit to being so. The threesome scene therefore can often provide an opportunity for those Geminis who want to openly express their bisexuality.

The Gemini woman, who is outwardly rather prim and proper, can really let her hair down when she is inspired to do so. She is in fact one of the sexiest of all the star signs.

The studious Gemini male will abandon his books and turn into a hot blooded lover when between the sheets.

If the Gemini male uses condoms he will have a twin pack nearby.

Both male and female Geminis like explicit sex talk when making love.

CANCER June 22nd to July 23rd

Cancer's element is water.

Cancerians have a very healthy appetite for sex but love has to come first. They are sentimental and thoughtful lovers who will take time to please a partner. They need plenty of encouragement before introducing anything new to their sex lives.

Cancerians are turned on by soft pornography and raunchy books.

The Cancerian male can worry about sex and will abstain if he lacks confidence. If he uses condoms he will choose the kind that cling.

LEO July 24th to August 23rd

Leo is a fire sign.

Leos love sex. They are ardent, dramatic and very confident lovers - but they are fussy.

Leos like comfort and luxury and only like to make love in comfortable places. Once they are in their comfort zone and enjoying sex they like to talk in graphic sexual terms.

When making love the Leo female stimulates her man by giving every part of his body her attention.

The Leo male has a reputation for being the perfect lover. He will take his time and know just the right places to touch to satisfy his partner. His condoms tend to be flamboyant and come in one size only – large.

VIRGO August 24th to September 23rd

Virgo is an earth sign.

Both Virgo men and women are highly sexed. Their symbol is an earth sign and they start having sex early in their lives. They like to be in control of their sexual activities which can be varied. Many are bondage devotees and Virgo women like to role play and act out their sexual fantasies.

Virgo men are very conscious of health risks so they are unlikely to forget to wear a condom. Virgos tend anyway to be obsessive about personal hygiene.

Because love and sex are separate issues for Virgos they can be unfaithful.

They have no problem with indulging in sex outside a partnership. Virgos often become swingers which is a perfect way for them to have sex without emotional attachments.

Virgos will be the first to choose condoms that are environmentally friendly when some enterprising company starts making the biodegradable kind. Perhaps someone from such a company will read this and take the hint.

LIBRA September 24th to October 23rd

Libra's element is air.

Lovemaking is very important to Librans who often confuse sex with love. Members of this star sign do not like quickies and prefer quality over quantity.

Librans, with a tendency to laziness, love sex when it takes little physical effort.

The Libran female may not make love often but when she does it has to be just right.

The Libran male has a psychic intuition about what pleases a woman. He is very good at giving his partner an erotic massage and oral sex. He will choose the sensual condom that is mutually pleasing.

SCORPIO October 24th to November 22nd

Scorpio, whose element is water, is a very sensitive sign and perhaps sexually contradictory because Scorpios can be quite shy and a little prudish but also very sexual.

In the latter case for example the Scorpio woman can be a very exotic lover once she trusts her man.

The Scorpio male likes striptease and he appreciates his woman wearing good quality underwear.

Scorpios are risk takers and neither the male nor the female Scorpio like using condoms.

SAGITTARIUS November 23rd to December 21st

Members of this fire sign have a roving eye and can be sexually restless. Staying faithful to a partner therefore is very difficult. They are open-minded and interested in kinky sex.

Sagittarians like quickies whether indoors or out. They often have casual sex with friends and strangers.

The Sagittarian male, conscious of safe sex, will always wear an extra thick condom.

CAPRICORN December 22nd to January 20th

Capricorns, whose element is earth, need to be in secure relationships before they can enjoy sex. They can be inhibited unless they are with the right partner to bring out their earthy sexuality. They will try out new sexual positions with the aid of a text book – a practice which appeals to their dry sense of humour.

Capricorn females blossom sexually with an attentive partner.

The Capricorn male often feels under pressure to perform sexually which can lead to problems. He will choose the most traditional and durable type of condom.

AQUARIUS January 21st to February 19th

Aquarians, whose element is air, are two different types where sexual attitudes are concerned. The first type adopts a take it or leave it approach. For this Aquarian, sex is just a physical release. The other Aquarian likes to express the spiritual aspect of sex and will get involved with Tantric or magickal sex. However, both types can often find sexual gratification through fetishism.

The Aquarian male will choose the kinkier condoms – often going for bright colours and unusual shapes.

PISCES February 20th to March 20th

Pisces is a water sign.

Pisceans are romantic and sexually very active. This star sign can be a bit too imaginative for straight sex. It is not surprising, when you think of their star symbol, that Pisceans like making love in water.

The Piscean woman loves all forms of sex and she will encourage her partner to try out new ways of enjoying sex. Jean Harlow was a typical Piscean.

The Piscean male encourages his woman to wear sexy underwear. He likes sex toys and will think nothing of buying one as a gift for his partner. He will choose extra sensitive condoms and the kind that are spiked.

Section 6
Not a Lot of People Know

1

Menstruation
and the Moon

I am often asked, "Why is it that women are more psychic than men?" The simple answer is because women bleed.

Almost every woman becomes incredibly psychic and sensitive around the time of her period. Many women find that they have intuitive dreams when they are menstruating – and menstruation is one of the few things that really make women different from men.

Magickally, it is beneficial for women to talk to the Moon. Talking to the Moon should ease any period problems or difficulties. By period problems I mean of course the usual discomforts suffered by many. Do see your doctor though if you experience any untoward or uncharacteristic symptoms during your time of the month.

Our ancient ancestors knew that menstruation and the Moon's cycle go hand in hand. The Moon is a symbol of renewal with its own regular cycle.

A full Moon is associated with ovulation and the dark of the Moon is associated with menstruation. Some females notice that their cycles start at the full Moon or the dark of the Moon but never at the quarter Moon.

The Romans called the calculation of time menstruation. At one time the lunar calendars all had 28 day months. The four 7 day weeks within any month marked the new, waxing, full and waning Moon.

Every month the Moon grows until it reaches its full size and then shrinks again. This is where women's cycles are similar to that of the Moon. In fact, long ago all women menstruated at the same time because they were connected to the natural rhythms of the Moon and earth. It was with the introduction of electricity and the constant bombardment of artificial light that women's cycles began to change.

Studies have shown that women who for example have sex once a week experience normal menstrual cycles and a milder menopause. This is in comparison to women who have irregular sex or who are celibate.

Even today, menstruation is rarely talked about. Sadly, many attitudes about menstruation are still influenced by several negative aspects of old cultures, for example, in some aboriginal tribes, men believed that death would come if they came into contact with anything that had been touched by a menstruating woman. Even the sight of a menstruating female was considered to be dangerous.

Christian writers in the seventeenth century insisted that old women were filled with magick power because their menstrual blood remained in their veins.

The Orthodox Jewish religion forbids a married couple to touch from the moment a spot of blood appears at the onset of the woman's period until a week after menstruation has ceased.

With a variety of taboos still connected to menstruation, it is no wonder that women feel guilty about having sexual feelings during their periods. The fact is that many women continue to be sexually aroused at this time of the month. Sex is a wonderful relaxant and can help with period cramps. Yes, sex can be messy at this time, so the appropriate preparation is required such as a rubber sheet or towel placed underneath the woman.

Moon energy is called upon by witches for the casting of spells, so a woman's Moon time is ideal for performing magick rituals.

In contrast to examples of the past and present taboos that I have mentioned, members of the Hell's Angels "bikers" are said to earn their red wings by having oral sex with a woman who is on her period.

Someone who is sexually stimulated by underwear that has been worn by a menstruating woman is called a hematolagniac. These soiled items of clothing will be used as a focus for masturbation. Hematolagnia is a category of sexual behaviour that moves into the area of vampirism.

Another act of menstrual sex play is called "rainbow kissing", performed by having menstrual blood in the mouth. This is one of the customs of those who call themselves vampires.

2

The Secret Woman in Some Men's Lives: the Last Taboo

In 1992 the movie *Just Like a Woman* was released in the UK. The film starred Julie Walters and Adrian Pasdar. What made this film unusual was that transvestism was the theme of the story; a difficult subject to present on screen to the general public.

Just Like a Woman was premiered in the West End of London with Princess Diana attending. Also in attendance at the cinema to welcome Diana were some male members of a well-known transvestite and transsexual counselling group. All the group members at the premiere were fully dressed and made-up as females.

The movie's story is taken from a book entitled *Geraldine – For the Love of a Transvestite – an autobiographical episode.* The "autobiographical episode" is the sensitively written record of authoress Monica Jay's love affair with a cross-dresser named Gerald.

A significant fact in the story is that Gerald, who becomes Geraldine when dressed as a woman, is heterosexual.

A sexually straight cross-dresser no doubt sounds like a contradiction to many who believe that transvestites are gay, but the majority of cross-dressers are in fact heterosexual. And, within that majority, a high proportion of them are married or have female partners.

At the time that *Just Like a Woman* was released in 1992, it was quoted in the media that, "one in every hundred males is a transvestite." Whether that statistic was accurate or not, the reality is that a considerable number of men cross-dress. This fact is borne out by the magazines, books, specialist clothing outlets and clubs that cater to transvestites and transsexuals in the UK. This transgender industry is also evident to a greater or lesser degree throughout Europe, America and other countries.

To enter the world of the transvestite (the word transvestite originates from the German *transvestit*, literally meaning cross-dresser), it is necessary to start with the cross-dresser's childhood.

The first hint of transvestism can begin in a boy as young as four, five or six years old. At that early age of development he may already be showing signs of interest in female underwear, outerwear and make-up.

Significantly, many transvestites are brought-up in an all female environment without a male role model. This of course is ideal for the young embryo cross-dresser, whose mother will probably be more tolerant than a father would be of a son's fascination with all things female. She is also likely to regard her son's interest as a passing phase.

This phase does not pass, and, as the child reaches puberty and beyond, his need to cross-dress increases and intensifies. His transvestism is now an essential and often controlling part of his life.

Transvestism, also known as the "last taboo", can exact a heavy price for the cross-dresser who can lose his wife, family and friends because they are unable to accept a man who wants to be – just like a woman.

The sad twist in the tale of the transvestite is that in expressing his feminine side, he is frequently misunderstood by a member of the gender he most admires – a female.

The average unaware cross-dresser's wife or partner is likely to react with horror and dismay when she first catches her man clad in silky lingerie and stockings. Is he gay? Is he on the verge of wanting a sex change operation? These are the first questions that the partner will be asking.

The belief that transvestites are gay no doubt stems in part from the fact that a great number of drag artists are homosexual. But these artists perform in drag as a profession. In the main they do not dress up as females because they have an emotional need to do so.

Transsexuals, in comparison with transvestites, are few. The pre operation transsexual typically feels like "a woman trapped in a man's body", which is not the mindset of the cross-dresser.

Transvestites will often fantasize about being biologically female – but they would miss the sexual side of being male if they had a sex change operation.

A TV, to use the abbreviation, is often sexually attracted to an older woman, particularly if the older woman is sympathetic to his cross-dressing. This preference can be linked back to the TV's childhood where the dominant influence was likely to have been an older woman such as the boy's mother or grandmother – or both. And "dominant" is another key to the cross-dresser's sexuality because he often likes to be sexually submissive to a dominant female.

The transvestite, particularly in his early life, is also sexually stimulated by wearing female clothing, especially very feminine silky underwear, stockings and satin faced foundation wear; so there is a strong fetish element to the TV's sexual persona.

The true TV is at his happiest when fully dressed and made-up as a female. This is the time when he can express his soft, feminine side – and bring out the woman who is always within. For many TVs the woman within has to remain a secret woman.

Several of my friends are cross-dressers so I have a unique insight into their world. It is a world that embraces and expresses the feminine whilst retaining the masculine. Confusing? Yes. It can be very confusing and contradictory to outsiders, but less so to some of the women who know about their partners' cross-dressing. Here are some composite comments that come from those women who accept their men's feminine side:

Not only do I have a husband but I have a girlfriend too.

I would rather know about his cross-dressing than have him lead a secret life that I can't share.

He's more sensitive when he's dressed as a female and expressing his feminine side.

His hobby doesn't involve anyone else and does no harm at all.

It's great fun for us to go shopping together for women's clothes.

We have a wonderful, loving relationship. Why should I worry about his cross-dressing?

Such statements from tolerant TVs' partners make a refreshing change to the ignorant prejudice that is suffered by so many cross-dressers.

Luckily, in the UK, we have the well established *Beaumont Society* and *The Gender Trust*. These charities help respectively TVs and TVs' partners. Contact details for these organizations will be found in *Miscellaneous Information*.

There are also a number of other counselling groups in the UK, many of them mentioned and listed in the *Transgender A to Z*. This annual publication, known as the "Bible of the Transgendered World", covers the UK and international transgender scene with extensive club and contact information.

In this chapter I have of necessity generalized to a certain degree about cross-dressing and the cross-dresser because of space limitation. Nevertheless, I do feel that I have given you a good background picture of a very complex subject. In turn, I hope that those of you who may be suspicious of transvestism will now have a more understanding and sympathetic view of the cross-dresser.

3
The Sexual Aspects of Essential Oils

Most people identify essential oils with aromatherapy but these magickal and mystical natural plant essences have other uses. They also have their individual sexual and romantic aspects.

Ten essential oils and their sexual associations, together with guidance on how to use the oils, are given below:

Caraway *(Carum carvi)*

To attract a lover, you should mentally write your own short love story, with yourself as a warm, emotional person giving and receiving love. Use caraway oil in a burner to add to your mood and aid your romantic visualization.

Lovers who have argued can smooth out their problems by burning this oil.

Carnation *(Dianthus caryothyllus)*

The carnation is known as the flower of Zeus. The oil of this flower is said to bring spicy love-making to your sex life.

Ginger *(Zingiber officinalis)*

Inhaling the fragrance of ginger is believed to stimulate your physical body, generating exciting muscular contraction and bioelectrical energy – which is the electricity generated by the body.

The spicy scent of ginger has long been used to create sexual desire.

Jasmine (Jasminum officinale)

This exotic fragrance is used worldwide to create the necessary emotional and physical responses for sexual arousal.

Jasmine is also used to help women and men with sexual problems. For example, women who find it hard to achieve orgasm or pleasure from sex, and men with erection problems, could be helped by sniffing this fragrance whilst visualizing making love.

Neroli (Citrus aurantium)

Neroli is a heady rich scent which has a tradition for alleviating worry about sexual performance. This fragrance also helps to harmonize sexual relationships.

Patchouli (Pogostemon cablin)

The scent of patchouli is often employed to help arouse sexual desire.

This fragrance is believed to banish sexual anxiety and prepare its users for exciting sexual experiences.

An added bonus with patchouli is that it can be used in a magickal context to manifest money when funds are low.

Rose (Rosa)

The scent of roses turns our thoughts to love, on top of which, roses act as an aphrodisiac, influencing the brain and sexual centres of the body.

Roses are also associated with alleviating female sexual problems, and the scent of this flower is helpful in overcoming psychological impotence in the male.

Sandalwood (Santalum album)

Sandalwood, universally popular in the form of incense sticks and pleasantly perfumed toilet items, can be used to help those suffering from impotence and emotional frigidity.

Sandalwood has a strong tradition as an aphrodisiac. A few drops of sandalwood oil in the bath could bring pleasing results.

Vanilla *(Vanilla aromatica and vanilla planifolia)*

In American folk magick, women traditionally place a few drops of vanilla tincture behind their ears to attract men.

Vanilla has a warm aroma that is said to trigger sexual desire and can be used to arouse either the male or the female!

Ylang Ylang *(Cananga odorata)*

Ylang ylang has an incredibly erotic fragrance. This oil is said to dilute anger, have a calming effect, eradicate a negative emotional state, create sexual desire – and bring love into your life.

I have given you details of ten oils but there are over one hundred and forty oils listed in essential oil supplier *Tree-harvest's* catalogue. So you can see that you are spoilt for choice.

When buying essential oils it is very important that you obtain pure oils and not the synthetic variety. Only pure plant essences have the unique quality that is an absolute must for magickal work. If in doubt contact *Tree-harvest, Neal's Yard* or *Baldwin* who are suppliers of good plant oils.

There are various ways in which to use essential oils. You can add half a dozen drops to your bath water; evaporate the oil in a purpose made burner, or use the oil as a scent in a cologne preparation.

I wish you many magickal moments with these mystical plant essences.

4

No Smoke without Fetish

Between the 1920s and 1940s, we saw film stars like Marlene Dietrich and Veronica Lake puffing seductively on cigarettes.

Actresses smoking on screen at that time were often playing women of easy virtue and the cigarette accentuated that image. Also, if we look at that period in the history of cinema, overt sex was never expressed on the silver screen. Smoking a cigarette though suggested that sex was about to take place or had taken place.

Pornographic photographs from the 1930s era would often show naked women smoking cigarettes or with cigarettes in their vaginas. The cigarette was and is a phallic symbol.

Some cigarette fetishists are attracted to women who smoke long cigarettes. Others are attracted to those who smoke white or brown tipped cigarettes.

A man with a cigarette smoking fetish thinks that a woman who smokes is self-confident and sophisticated. But just as attractive to him can be the virginal looking woman who smokes. He can also be really aroused by the phallic shape of a cigarette held between a woman's high glossed red lips - and the overall sexual turn on is a long cigarette holder held between those same glossy red lips.

Bright red lipstick was the fashion in the 1940s and any cigarette fetishist with a penchant for red lipstick will insist that this colour is worn by the woman who is smoking for his sexual pleasure.

I have often thought that many of those with a smoking fetish could be bringing through a strong echo from past lives lived up to and through the 1940s. Those years were in many ways the start of a social liberation when smoking was popular and women smoked openly in public.

Smoke is an important part of the cigarette fetish, from the turn-on of seeing a woman exhaling smoke through her nostrils to blowing smoke rings. Many men also enjoy having their partners blow smoke over their genitals before or during oral sex.

Amanda, who was a client of mine, had a partner with a smoking fetish. Both of them smoked but she suffered from high blood pressure. She had been told quite bluntly by her doctor that she risked having a stroke unless she stopped smoking. Her self-centred partner was not sympathetic and encouraged her to continue smoking. He liked to blow smoke over her genitals and she did the same to him. This entrenched sexual ritual made it very difficult for Amanda to kick her smoking habit.

A fetish such as this, which is attached to an addiction, is a hard habit to break, but I do advise you to try to stop smoking if you are in a situation like Amanda's. There are addiction counsellors to contact and many products on the market to help you do this. Ask your doctor or local *Boots* or *Superdrug* store for advice. Alternatively, cut out smoking in stages by using tar reducing disposable filters such as *Super 25*. See the *Appendix* for details.

I have no problem at all with folk who are having their own kind of sex fun but it should not endanger health - particularly a partner's health. Enjoy your sex in safe ways.

5

Body Piercing Sex Magick

Witches have known for centuries that genital piercing can turn the most frigid woman into a sex goddess. Over the years I have suggested many different techniques to help women deal with a low sex drive. One of my recommended techniques is body piercing with an appropriate metal adornment. Also in this chapter are other aspects of body piercing sex magick for both genders.

When I give advice and tips about body piercing in this chapter, take it as read that I am talking about the attachment of metal adornments in pierced flesh.

Clitoris hood

For those who are game enough to try it, piercing the clitoris hood is in the top ten of effective treatments.

Many women, after having their clitoris hood pierced, are able to have an orgasm just by walking in a certain way.

Ear lobes

Ears are sexy and earlobes are sexually sensitive, yet ears are pierced more today for the adornment of earrings.

However, in some ancient cultures, ears were pierced to stop demons entering the body through the ears. It was thought that metal and metal earrings repelled these entities and stopped them gaining access to the body. Some societies also pierced ears as part of a puberty ritual.

Nipples

For both men and women there are numerous benefits to be had by having nipples pierced, such as making small nipples look larger.

Nipples are also more sensitive and sexually attractive when pierced – and the problem of inverted nipples can also be dealt with by piercing.

Nose

Nose piercing was recorded over four thousand years ago in the Middle East. This practice was even mentioned in the Bible's Book of Genesis.

Nose piercing is thought to accentuate the face and make it sexier and the artistic genius Leonardo da Vinci felt that a person's nose expressed their character.

Penis

A man will find that his penis becomes more sensitive after piercing. Piercing is done through the little flap of skin just below the head of the penis.

Tongue

The Aztecs were one of many ancient civilizations that engaged in tongue piercing. This Amerindian culture believed that blood drawn from tongue piercing allowed their holy men to go into an altered state of consciousness so that they could commune with the Gods.

Women and men who like oral sex find that a stud in the tongue improves cunnilingus and fellatio.

A cautionary note

If you are thinking of having body piercing, it is advisable to go to a recognized parlour. Preferably, choose an establishment that has been recommended by a reliable source.

6

Historical Facts about Sex Aids and Toys

Clitoral stimulator

The clitoral stimulator originates from ancient China. This device started as a carved ivory ring that was put on a man's penis to maintain his erection. Over a period of time the ring evolved in design to incorporate a nub that would rub against a woman's clitoris, so giving her more pleasure during sexual intercourse.

Cock ring

The cock ring is another accessory that comes from ancient China. The first records of cock rings tell us that they were made from the eyelids of goats with the animals' eyelashes intact. The flexible eyelids were placed around a man's erection and the lashes were said to increase the woman's sexual enjoyment.

Dildo

The first dildos appeared circa 500 BC. They originated from Greece - and Mediterranean traders sold them as sex toys for lonely women.

Love ball

The love ball was invented around 500 AD. The love ball was originally used to increase a man's sexual pleasure during intercourse. Some of the balls were solid but others were hollow with clappers that made a ringing sound as they rolled around in a woman's vagina. In time the balls were paired and used by a woman to strengthen her pelvic floor muscles.

Lubricant

Couples were using olive oil as a sexual lubricant circa 500 BC. Since that time, a variety of natural vegetable oils have been used for the same purpose.

Mirror

Circa 655 AD saw the introduction of the mirror as a sexual accessory.

The Chinese emperor Tai Tsung's consort had sheets of reflecting glass arranged around their bed. These sheets were later removed when she was advised that, according to feng shui, mirrors placed in such a position are a bad omen.

In the *Sex Magick* chapter I too warn against mirrors at the side or bottom of a shared bed because this positioning is not good for a relationship.

Penis extension

The first penis extenders, now known as prosthetic penis attachments, appeared in 200 AD. This device would fit over a man's erection to make his penis look larger. They were made from wood, leather, animal horn, ivory and metal – including gold and silver.

Penis extenders were first mentioned in such sex manuals as the *Kama Sutra*.

Polaroid Land Camera

The Polaroid Land Camera arrived on the photographic scene in 1948. With an instant photo developing facility, this camera was a boon to the amateur pornographer who could take and then privately develop pornographic and erotic pictures within minutes.

Rubber

In 1844 vulcanized rubber was used to make strong rubber dildos and other sex aids. The development of latex rubber products started about 1930.

Lighter and softer than vulcanised rubber, latex was ideal for the manufacture of condoms and diaphragms.

Vibrator:)

And now we come to probably the most popular sex toy of all time – in all its many variations.

The first vibrator was invented by an American physician George Taylor MD. The year was 1869, four years after the American civil war ended. Taylor's vibrator was a large, awkward, steam powered device. The doctor recommended his invention for the treatment of what was known at the time as female hysteria. This of course was a cover term for the emotional and physical symptoms of female frustration and sexual arousal. In the Victorian period women were not considered to be sexually aware so their "hysteria" had to be treated as an illness. Doctors of the time treated this condition by massaging the sufferers' vulvas until they reached orgasm. This of course encouraged more hysteria and the women needed more treatments.

In 1899 America's first electric vibrator was mentioned in a periodical. This vibrator was advertised as a cure for headaches, wrinkles and nerve pain.

In 1921 men were being encouraged to buy their wives vibrators for Christmas. It was said that vibrators would keep them young, wrinkle free and – here we go again – free from the menace of hysteria.

In 1952 the medical profession decided that the time was right to finally declare that hysteria was not a real health ailment. From then on the vibrator's true and unambiguous function was acknowledged and it was, and is, sold today under its true colours as a sex accessory.

Coming up to date, we now have the famous rabbit vibrator which was shown in the popular 1998 television series *Sex and the City*. After this kind of exposure, sales of the rabbit vibrator went through the roof.

Today, vibrators are made from a range of different materials and they are available in different sizes, shapes and colour finishes.

Water bed

The water bed made its debut in 1970. Inventor Charles P Hall had a comfortable sleep in mind for his prospective customers when he designed his water bed but it soon gained a reputation for providing a new sexual experience.

Playboy magazine proprietor Hugh Hefner soon had a water bed installed at his Chicago Playboy mansion and many hotels followed his lead by having them added to their honeymoon suites.

Whip

The whip has always had a strong sexual association, primarily with the practice of flagellation.

The first brothels providing a flagellation service, along with other sadomasochistic activities, were recorded in 1750.

Today, the dominatrix who provides a flagellation service will often have on her card a name such as "Miss Whiplash", thereby leaving no doubt as to what her speciality is.

7

Playing
with Fire

Apart from keeping us warm and cooking our food, fire allied with magick has often gone hand in hand, whether for use in fertility and sacrificial rites in the distant past to the timeless practice of fire and flame divination.

Fire also has a more secretive aspect for it is obviously the essential element for sadomasochists who like to play with fire in the literal, sexual sense.

A few years ago I was invited to give some Tarot readings at an S & M sex club in Bristol which had a fire dominatrix demonstrating her speciality. I took with me my set of erotic Tarot cards, which I thought very appropriate for this particular club.

It had been a pleasant journey by road from Leicestershire to Bristol and I took the last available parking space outside the club. I had taken the precaution of visualizing a parking space before arriving.

The double black fire doors were open as I walked through into the club's interior with my reading table and cards. Other psychics and exhibitors were arriving too and carrying their goods in.

As I adjusted my sight to the interior's darkness I could see that I was in what looked like a cave with niches full of clothes racks displaying every kind of fetish gear.

I found my space at one side of the stage on which the fire dominatrix would be demonstrating and set up my reading table. Then with time to spare I wandered around the stalls which had every kind of S & M accessory for sale including handcuffs, corsets and whips. There were even teddy bears dressed in all kinds of bondage outfits.

Once the club doors were open to its members it was not long before my first client walked over. He was a thin, tall man dressed in a long coat. Before he sat down at my table he asked me if he could open his coat. "Of course" I said, so he opened his coat wide to reveal his nakedness. His action was quite unexpected but this after all was not a "normal" club. He asked me if I could see his penis and I said that I could. My answer seemed to relax him and with that formality out of the way I asked him to shuffle the Tarot cards.

The cards revealed that there was a woman and two children with this man. He admitted that he was married and had a son and daughter. I also saw him walking naked in public, a very dangerous thing to do. The cards also indicated a shock in store and that a warning should be given so I advised him to restrict his exhibitionism to the premises we were in - or join a nudist club. He admitted that he had recently been taking some silly risks and promised to heed my advice.

I gave one more Tarot reading before the club's 1.55 pm deadline, after which the fire dominatrix would take centre stage for her demonstration at 2.00 pm.

The dominatrix appeared exactly on time. She had short brown hair and was dressed in a tight blue and black rubber dress that accentuated her amazing figure. The dress was zipped in the front in such a way that she could display some cleavage. She was extremely pretty and had a lovely smiling face.

The dominatrix looked out beyond the stage and asked for a volunteer to help her with her act.

A young man appeared who I recognized as one of the club's slave helpers. He was about 20 and wore blue jeans and a grey T-shirt.

The dominatrix ushered him up onto the stage and asked him to remove his outer clothes. He hastily stripped down to a woman's pair of pink frilly panties which he kept on.

The dominatrix then took her volunteer over to a giant cross and attached his wrists and ankles to leather straps which were secured to the large structure.

With her volunteer restrained, the dominatrix next lit a torch which looked like the type that a circus fire eater would use. Carefully guiding the torch, she ran the flames over the young man's chest then down his arms and legs. Apart from a few small gasps he never flinched.

The aroma of his singed body hairs came across from the stage and stayed in the air long after the demonstration had ended. This had been a most unusual and at the same time fascinating demonstration of sex play with fire.

After the stage act was over I made a point of asking the young volunteer if he had been hurt or felt any pain.

He told me that he had suffered no pain but he had enjoyed the fantastic experience.

Other kinds of associated sex play include lighting a candle and dripping the melting wax over the body of a willing partner.

At the beginning of this chapter I mentioned fire and flame divination which is known as pyromancy. Here are a few interpretations to start you off if you want to try your hand at reading fires.

A good future lies ahead for anyone whose fire burns quickly.

Success on the way is indicated by clear red flames.

Obstacles are shown by dull yellow flames.

An envious person wanting to harm you is the warning given by a constantly spitting fire.

Confusion around you is shown by flames blowing in the wind.

Reach for the sky when the smoke from a fire ascends without a change in direction.

Difficult times ahead are shown by a fire that is difficult to light or slow to burn.

Let me now add an obvious but necessary cautionary note. Whether you are barbecuing, lighting stoves, fires or candles, fire can be dangerous to your health and safety. Please be careful with naked fire and flames because there is nothing more horrific than an accident or death by burning.

8

The French Courtesan and Count Dracula's Protégé

In this, the last of the *Not a Lot of People Know* chapters, the following true account of possession was known to no more than half a dozen people of whom I was one. The reason why this story has been kept secret by the couple concerned will become apparent.

Many years ago I had a friend named Jane who I first met with her husband David at a psychic fayre. The three of us were chatting one day about occult matters when I mentioned vampires. At this point Jane quickly asked me to change the subject. My curiosity was aroused and I asked Jane why she wanted to avoid the subject. As she hesitated, I pressed her again to tell me why. Eventually she told me. Her story, which I retell here is quite frightening, even more so because it is true.

Jane was 18 years old and a Cambridge student when she suffered the first of a number of frightening spirit possessions.

It all started when she went out with a couple of friends for what began as a normal, relaxed, girly evening out; a round of drinks in a wine bar followed by a visit to a nightclub.

After leaving the wine bar where they had spent the early part of the evening, the young women walked to the club. As soon as they were inside they found a table and Jane went to the bar to get their drinks. Sitting at the bar was a man who started speaking to her in French.

Jane, who was unable to understand what he was saying because she did not speak French, just smiled politely and walked away with her drinks.

Jane returned to her table where she sat with her friends for the next hour when suddenly she had the sensation of someone, or something, climbing into her body. What happened next was that she found the Frenchman standing by her side.

He introduced himself to Jane by giving a name that sounded to her like Mattu. It is most likely that he was giving the French name Mathieu. Then to Jane's total astonishment she found that she was speaking to the man in fluent French.

The Frenchman's conversation became overtly sexual towards her and she found herself telling him that she was a courtesan and that her services would cost him x amount of francs.

Without further discussion Mathieu accepted her fee and asked her to accompany him to his lodging room. She agreed to go with him and they walked out of the club together.

From that moment Jane was unable to recollect what happened to her on that night or how she got home.

When Jane got out of bed in the morning she found that she was totally naked. This was very strange because she always wore a nightdress – she never ever slept in the nude. And, when she caught sight of herself in the wardrobe mirror, something even stranger, she saw that she had puncture marks on her neck, breasts and thighs.

Jane, now in a worried state, rang her friends to ask them what they could remember of their evening out. They both told Jane that she had left the club without collecting her coat or saying goodbye to them. Neither of the two young women recalled seeing their friend leave with any man.

Jane knew that if her strange experience had only happened once she could have put it down to having consumed too much alcohol.

However, the spirit of the French courtesan who had possessed her on that evening took over her body frequently over a period of many years.

Jane got married and through the years her husband David had on numerous occasions witnessed Jane's transformation into the French courtesan, complete with the ability to speak fluent French.

Jokingly, when Jane first shared her story with me, I had asked her if the puncture marks were put there by Count Dracula's French protégé but neither she nor David laughed. They both told me that they never talked about the problem because if they did, "then bad things happen." Jane said to me, "If we speak about vampires a dark entity is drawn towards both of us."

At first I could not help looking for a *Candid Camera* wind-up behind Jane's story, even though her tale was confirmed and added to by David. It was not long though before I realized that their strange account was not only genuine but they were both very afraid too.

I lost touch with them until years later when I was working at a Cambridge psychic fayre. Halfway through the morning I saw a familiar face as Jane walked up to my table.

It was good to see her again after the passage of time. She told me that she had got a lot to tell me and asked me to go and have a coffee with her.

Over lunchtime coffees we reminisced and Jane related that the French courtesan had continued to control her.

Jane said that eventually she had sought help from a Wiccan High Priestess in the north of England. The witch told her she was possessed by an eighteenth century high class prostitute who had been sadistically murdered by having the blood drained from her body.

The High Priestess then performed an exorcism on Jane and placed a blessing on David.

However, several questions remained unanswered …

Was the Frenchman that Jane met at the bar the spirit of the sadistic murderer who killed the courtesan by draining her body of blood?

Was the Frenchman just a tourist passing through Cambridge?

Was the Frenchman in fact a vampire? Ah, you may laugh - but read on.

Why did Jane's husband David often wake-up to find puncture marks on **his** body too?

Not a lot of people will know the answers to these questions – probably only two, the French courtesan and her fellow countryman.

Section 7
Conclusion
and Information

During my involvement in the occult world over a forty-five year period I have worked, met and socialized with astrologers, Spiritualists, witches, a Zambian medicine man, a Native American medicine man and a very gifted magickal artist. Many in this large group are close friends. Never though had I ever come across a witch specializing in human sexual behaviour before I came into contact with Dr Tarona Hawkins.

I have learned much through my association with Tarona Hawkins which emphasizes the point that no matter what your age, you can always add something new to your knowledge bank. This has certainly been the case for me as I have gone through the vast amount of material that has come my way through working with this amazing witch.

After long months of writing, interspersed with countless telephone conversations talking to Tarona, this volume materialized. My input on the project was intended to give Tarona more time to herself but inevitably, as the book progressed and evolved, we established a continuous communication.

I liked Tarona's philosophy from the beginning for she made and makes a point of never moralizing with her sex counselling except to say that one's actions should harm none. She also gives specific cautions from time to time that are relevant to the subject under discussion.

I want to repeat here what I said in the *Introduction* to this book which is that *Secrets of the Sex Witch* will be the most unusual sex handbook that you have ever read. As you reach the end of this book, I think you will agree that you have been reading something that is quite different from anything else in the witchcraft and sex handbook categories.

I suspect that there will be some who will try to copy the style and content of *A WITCH'S GUIDE* - but a copy is just that - and a counterfeit will never ever have the same impact as an original.

A WITCH'S GUIDE contains some heavy subject matter in places so Tarona and I thought that it would be good to lighten-up and close with some of her hilarious personal stories. The following anecdotes are tales from her years working as a psychic and sex witch. I invite you to relax with me and enjoy some humour therapy!

Howard Rodway

You must be psychic

As I waited at my reading table for my first client to arrive at the psychic fayre, I was aware of a Spiritualist medium sitting to my left. He was totally engrossed in the reading he was giving to the person opposite him who hung on every word that he said.

To my right was a space reserved for a blonde psychic who had just arrived. The first thing she did before setting up her table was to plug in her electric kettle at a point low down on the wall behind the medium.

The medium, continuing with his reading, was now in communication with a soul who had passed over. At this stage the spiritualist's intent sitter, who was looking at a misty cloud rising in front of her, exclaimed in an excited voice, "I can see spirit."

"Can you?" responded the medium, "You must be psychic."

It was then that I felt that it only correct to interrupt and tell them that the spirit was no more than the steam rising from the kettle which had given no warning whistle!

Bruno

The first psychic events at which I appeared were in Yorkshire and every Saturday and Sunday I would drive north to attend.

I love Yorkshire and its people who are straightforward, no-nonsense folk, but I was nevertheless delighted when the psychic event organiser suggested holding a fayre in my own home county of Leicestershire.

A day before the fayre was to take place I received a request from a Hull psychic asking me if I could put her up for the weekend. I happily agreed to do so.

My house guest from Hull arrived on the day before the fayre and my delightful dog Bruno ran to greet her at the door. Bruno was the most adorable canine in the world except that he had a wind problem.

During the weekend we, "we" being my husband and various friends, soon realized that the Hull psychic was obsessed with evil. In fact she was obsessed to the point of paranoia about the subject of dark forces and negative energy.

On the last evening that our house guest was with us, we had just finished eating our evening meal and we were all sitting around the table talking when Bruno, unobserved, walked over and crept under the dining room table for a spell of doggy meditation. As Bruno relaxed, his inside relaxed too, and an odour like swamp gas was released into the confined space of the dining room. The smell had nowhere to go but up and it soon enveloped all of us. Realising who was responsible for the emission, I was extremely embarrassed and apologized for Bruno's behaviour, adding that flatulence is unfortunately a characteristic of boxers.

My house guest, instead of accepting my apology and dismissing the incident so that we could move on, grabbed my hand, gazed into my eyes and gave me the filthiest of looks. She said, "So you think that's wind do you?"

"Of course," I replied.

"Well it's not, it's a psychic fart," she ranted.

"A what?" we all said in unison, trying not to laugh.

My obsessive guest replied, "A psychic fart. This dog is taking all the bad energy from you and that is why he is farting."

We all cracked up with laughter which did not go down too well with the lady from Hull who I suspected had a mental problem.

Needless to say, I never had this woman in my home again!

Sadly Bruno is no longer on the physical plane but the memory of that evening is one that will always be treasured.

The job description

Some years ago when I was a volunteer charity worker, part of my work involved visiting about seven brothels in my designated area to hand out condoms. The girls in these establishments were a marvellous source of extremely funny stories, but I also have my own firsthand account of house humour.

One day when I was on the "condom run" as I called it, I was in one particular brothel delivering the day's quota of condoms when I was privy to a conversation between the madam of the house and a young woman.

The owner was interviewing this young woman to see if she was suitable for the personal services that the establishment provided. The madam also had two of her girls sitting in on the interview.

The owner went into a detailed job description of the personal services that her establishment provided and added, "You will agree to do water sports won't you?"

The job applicant asked, "Water sports, so you have a swimming pool here do you?"

At this point, everyone including yours truly, started laughing, much to the bewilderment of the interviewee.

The owner quickly explained in specific terms what water sports were all about.

"Oh, I thought you meant water polo," said the girl.

I never saw this young woman again so I concluded that she never got the job.

Tarona Hawkins

About Dr Tarona Hawkins

Tarona Hawkins was born in Leicestershire, England, in 1950. Both her parents were born on witches' sabbat days, a fact that she believes has contributed to her strong psychic abilities.

Tarona Hawkins, a qualified hypnotherapist, past life regressionist, registered healer, medium, clairvoyant, doctor of metaphysics and a practising witch, is also a prolific writer who had her own paranormal *At the Edge* column in the *Loughborough and Shepshed Echo*. She has written numerous articles for American magazines and had her first book *Tarona's Ghostly Encounters* published by the Echo Press in 2000. In addition, she was the resident psychic for Loughborough's *107 Oak FM* radio station and she has appeared on several television programmes including the *Graham Norton Show*.

Dr Tarona's working day can involve investigating a haunted house, giving a hypnotherapy session, conducting a Tarot card reading and giving someone a telephone reading – such as she often gave to the late Princess Diana.

Increasingly over the years though, more and more of Tarona's clients have come to seek her help for their sex related problems.

As word has spread privately and publicly about her sex counselling and hypnotherapy treatments, she has become known as the *Sex Witch*, an unusual and unique title in the world of witches and witchcraft.

Dr Tarona Hawkins, who has a son and daughter, lives with her husband in East Anglia, England.

About Howard Rodway

Howard Rodway was born in Surrey, England, in 1936. He was educated at schools in Gloucestershire and the West Country. After completing his education, he left the United Kingdom for Zambia (then Northern Rhodesia). He spent some time in the Colonial Service, and he was a national serviceman in the Rhodesian Army. In 1958 he returned to Britain by signing on as a fireman aboard the Union Castle Line's *Drakensberg Castle*, a cargo-passenger vessel bound from Cape Town to London via the Suez Canal.

Soon after his arrival in the UK, he joined Government Communications Headquarters, where he stayed for a number of years.

Howard has been involved in the occult world since the sixties, during which time he has acted as a public relations manager for the late international clairvoyant Kim Tracey. He also represented the late Dr Fancis Ngombe, President of the Association of African and Asian Medicine Men.

Howard's psychic experiences have been related in *Psychic News* and in his first book *The Psychic Directory* (Futura, 1984). During 1986-1987 he wrote a series of articles about the occult for London's *Metropolitan* magazine. In December 1987, *The Stranger in the Snow*, a short story, was published in *Kent Life*. His other books are *Tarot of The Old Path* (Urania Verlag AG, 1990), *Tarot of Northern Shadows* (AGM AGMuller, 1998), *The Rune Vision Cards* (Vega, 2002), and also Swiss published English and German editions of *The Rune Vision Cards* (AGM AGMuller Urania 2008).

Miscellaneous Information

Aura photography

London based Paul Mitchell travels worldwide to demonstrate and take aura photographs. He also has an exhibition stand at the annual *Mind Body Spirit Festival* in London.
Website www.aurainternational.net
E-mail
paul@newpowersanctuary.com

Corsetry – lingerie – hosiery

Axfords
82 Centurion Road
Brighton
Sussex
BN1 3LN UK
Telephone 01273 327944
International dialling + 44 1273 327944
Website www.axfords.com
E-mail axfords@axfords.com

"Craft and quality hand made since 1880", is a statement of pride made by *Axfords* in their beautifully illustrated corsetry and foundation wear colour catalogue. *Axfords* internationally famous garments are hand crafted to very high standards. You can visit *Axfords* by arrangement to see these lovely corsets being made by hand. You can make an appointment by calling the number above and asking for the proprietor Mr Michael Hammond.

What Katie Did
Unit 8
The Old Mill
61 Reading Road
Pangbourne
Berkshire
RG8 7HY UK
Telephone 0845 4308743

International dialling + 44 845 4308743

Website www.whatkatiedid.com

What Katie Did – and does – is produce a stunning range of faux vintage glamour lingerie, most of which has been created by using original patterns. *Katie's* colour catalogue illustrates perfectly that the forties and fifties lingerie and hosiery was not only stylish but sexy too. You can also visit *What Katie Did's* boutique at:

Unit 26

Portobello Green

281 Portobello Road

London W10 5TZ

Telephone 0845 430 8943

International dialling +44 845 430 8943

Erotic art

Chris Francis BA FRSA UA

Website

www.artbychrisfrancis.co.uk

E-mail franciscomms@aol.com

Body portrait artist Chris Francis says, "Ladies – the sensual and sexy you, captured for posterity. Prolong your partner's enjoyment with an intimate portrait of your body – or that part of your body that really turns on your mate."

Chris is a member of the *Guild of Erotic Artists*.

Leigh Heppell

The Studios

Trenoweth

Mabe

Penryn

Cornwall

TR10 9JH UK

Telephone/fax 01326 376044

International dialling + 44 1326 376044

Erotic sculpture and body artist Leigh Heppell's exotic, sexually explicit sculptures have attracted clients from both the private and commercial sector. Leigh's work has also generated considerable comment in the conventional art world. All his sculptures are numbered limited editions and each work is supplied with a certificate of authentication.

Erotic Books

Bibliophile

Bibliophile Books

Unit 5 Datapoint Business Centre

South Crescent

London

E16 4TL UK

Telephone 0207 474 2474

International dialling + 44 207 474 2474

Website www.bibliophilebooks.com

E-mail orders@bibliophilebooks.com

Bibliophile has a justified reputation as the mail order market place in which to find bargains books. Amongst its many categories is the Erotica section, and within this section is *Bibliophile's* inner sanctum of erotica, *The Erotica Bookclub at www.curiosa.co.uk*

Taschen GMBH

Hohenzollernring 53

D-50672 Koln

Germany

International dialling telephone 00 49 221 201 800

Website www.taschen.com

This German publisher produces good quality and good value illustrated volumes of erotica which are prized by collectors. *Taschen* celebrated its twenty-fifth year in publishing in 2005 and now has global subsidiaries. *Taschen* invite you to stay informed about their new titles. You can request their magazine at www.taschen.com/magazine or write to them at the address above.

Essential oils

Tree-harvest

The Granary

Lintridge Farm

Bromsberrow Heath

Ledbury

Herefordshire

HR8 1PB UK

Telephone   01531   650764

International dialling + 44 1531 650764

Website www.tree-harvest.com

E-mail enquiries@tree-harvest.com

Tree-harvest carries an impressive range of essential oils and also stocks oil burners. Their range of worldwide resin incenses is impressive too. Howard particularly recommends their Greek Rose Incense for creating a magickal mood for that special occasion.

Geopathic Stress

British Society of Dowsers

Website www.britishdowsers.org/
Contact this society to find a local dowser to check your home for geopathic stress.

Health

Wholistic Health Direct

Unit 1
Five House Farm
Sandon Road
Therfield
Royston
Hertfordshire
SG8 9RE UK
Telephone   01763   284910
International dialling + 44 1763 284910
Website www.wholisticresearch.com
Wholistic Health Direct stock an impressive range of health related products such as air purifiers, seed, herb, grass and juice blenders, special diet products, enema kits, massagers, natural deodorants, pulsors, water distillers, *Medivac Microfilter* vacuum cleaners and yoga accessories.

Mini Filter Super 25

A1 Pharmaceuticals plc
Unit 3
Bessemer Park Industrial Estate
250 Milkwood Road
Herne Hill
London SE24 OHG
Telephone 020 7738 7373
International dialling
+ 44 20 7738 7373
Contact A1 Pharmaceuticals if you are unable to find *Super 25s* at your local tobacconist or chemist. These mini disposable filters are sold in packs of 10.

Herb seed suppliers

John Chambers
15 Westleigh Road
Barton Seagrave
Kettering
Northants
NN15 5AJ UK
Telephone   01933   652562
International dialling 1933 652562
This established mail order seed specialist, and winner of five gold medals for outdoor garden displays

at Chelsea Flower Shows, carries an excellent range of seeds for native and naturalised herbs together with seeds for grasses and wild flowers. *John Chambers* also stock books about herbs and herb gardening.

Suffolk Herbs Ltd
Monks Farm
Coggeshall Road
Kelvedon
Essex
CO5 9PG UK
Telephone 01376 572456
International dialling
+ 44 1376 572456
This established mail order seed company's catalogue lists a wide variety of native herb seeds and useful gardening accessories.

Personal hygiene

Corrymoor Mohair Socks
Corrymoor Farm
Stockland
Honiton
Devon
EX14 9DY UK
Telephone 01404 861245
International dialling + 44 1404 861245
Website www.corrymoor.com
E-mail socks@corrymoor.com
Nature has constructed mohair in such a way that this particular wool fibre will never give foot bacteria any room to thrive. Howard has worn *Corrymoor's* socks for years and he says they are the best treat his feet have ever had! *Corrymoor* stock a plain colour range for men, women and children.

The Deodorant Stone (UK) Ltd
Caer Delyn
Dolgran
Carmarthenshire
SA39 9BX UK
Telephone 01559 384856
International dialling
+ 44 1559 384856
Website:
www.deodorant-stone.co.uk
Deodorant Stone deodorants inhibit the formation of bacteria and are made from natural products. They do not contain harsh chemicals or aluminium chlorohydrate. The *Deodorant* Stone products are

cruelty free, non toxic and non staining.

Safe sex protection

C S Supplies
Southwick
Brighton
Sussex
BN42 4ZZ UK
Telephone 01273 593069
International dialling
+ 44 1273 593069
Website www.postalcondoms.co.uk
E-mail sales@postalcondoms.co.uk
C S Supplies stock a variety of branded condoms at wholesale prices for their worldwide customers. *C S Supplies* also have female condoms, lubricants and adult toys including rabbit vibrators.

M E Mail Order
P O Box 20
Biggleswade
Bedfordshire
SG18 0YA UK
Telephone 01767 601031
International dialling + 44 1767 601031
Website www.memailorder.com
E-mail sales@memailorder.com
M E Mail Order has in stock a variety of competitively priced condoms, sex toys and personal lubricants. Visit their website for details of the large range of products available.

Spiritualism

The Arthur Findlay College
Stansted Hall
Stansted
Essex
CM24 8UD UK
Website www.arthurfindlaycollege.org
Email: afc@snu.org.uk
Telephone 01279 813636
International dialling + 44 1279 813636
The focus of the *Arthur Findlay College* is to advance spiritual and psychic science. The College has a programme of lectures and also conducts healing and public services.

College of Psychic Studies

16 Queensberry Place

Kensington

London

SW7 2EB

Telephone 020 7589 3293

International dialling

+ 44 20 7589 3293

Website www.psychic-studies.org.uk

Emailcpstudies@aol.com

This psychic research centre offers a variety of lectures and courses. The *CPS* also has a library.

Spiritualist Association of Great Britain

33 Belgrave Square

London

SW1X 8QB

Telephone 020 7235 3351

International dialling

+ 44 20 7235 3351

This is a very familiar centre for spiritualists and known by them simply as *HQ*. Here you can attend talks, spiritualist services, have private readings with mediums and also have healing.

Transvestism and transsexualism

Beaumont Society

27 Old Gloucester Street

London

WC1N 3XX UK

24 hour information telephone 01582 412220 International dialling

+ 44 1582 412220

Website

www.beaumontsociety.org.uk

E-mail

enquiries@beaumontsociety.org.uk

This much respected organisation was started in 1966 as a self support group for transvestites, transsexuals and their partners and friends.

Beaumont Trust

BM Charity

London

WC1N 3XX UK

Telephone 07000 287878

International dialling + 44 7000 287878 (Tuesdays and Thursdays only from 7.00pm -11.00 pm)

Website http://

members@aol.com/bmonttrust

E-mail bmonttrust@aol.com

This educational charity has a help line on Tuesdays and Thursdays from 7.00pm till 11.00 pm, and also provides information and speakers to all who are interested in gender identity issues.

The Gender Trust

P O Box 3192
Brighton
Sussex
BN1 3WR UK
Telephone 01273 234024
International dialling + 44 1273 234024
Website www.gendertrust.com
E-mail gentrust@mistral.co.uk
This UK charity supports transsexuals, their families and partners. *The Gender Trust* produces a quarterly magazine, booklets, leaflets and information for employers and those professional bodies and individuals who are interested in gender identity issues.

Transgender A to Z

WayOut Publishing Co Ltd
P O Box 70
Enfield
EN1 2AE UK

24 hour information telephone 020 8363 0948 International dialling + 44 20 8363 0948
Website www.transgenderatoz.com
www.wayout-publishing.com
E-mail Vicky@wayout-publishing.com
The annual *Transgender A to Z* is not only a guide but a directory too, giving contact information for transvestite clubs and organizations worldwide. This publication also lists every kind of service catering to the transgendered community, together with personal stories and much more.

The WayOut Club

9 Crosswall (off Minories)
London
EC3 UK
Website www.thewayoutclub.com
Described as "The jewel in the crown of London's alternative night life," this is the weekend club for the transgendered plus their partners and friends. Members and non members are welcome. For more details of this friendly club with its floor shows, dancing and dining, see the club's website.

Witchcraft

The Pagan Federation

BM Box 7097

London

WC1 3XX

Website www.paganfed.demon.uk

Email:

Secretary@paganfed.demon.co.uk

Email (USA) Mthorn@aol.com

The Pagan Federation is a long standing recognized source of information on all aspects of witchcraft.

The Fellowship of Isis

Foundation Centre

Clonegal Castle

Enniscorthy

Irish Republic

Website www.fellowshipofisis.com

This international centre exists to recognize and bring together all those who follow a goddess philosophy so it is a particularly appropriate association for witches.

Bibliography

Adler, Margot – *Drawing Down the Moon* (Beacon Press, USA, 1986)

Barton, Blanche – *The Secret Life of a Satanist* (Feral House, USA, 1991)

Bourne, Lois – *Witch Amongst Us - the Autobiography of a Witch* (Robert Hale 1985)

Devi, Indra – *Yoga for You* (Thomas & Co., 1960)

Dunne, Desmond – *Yoga Made Easy* (Award Books, USA, 1966)

Farrar, Janet and Stewart – *The Witches' Goddess the Feminine Principle of Divinity* (Robert Hale, 1987)

Gurmukh – *The Eight Human Talents* (Thorsons, 2000)

Hawkins, Dr Tarona Gail – *Tarona's Ghostly Encounters* (Echo Press, 2000)

Jay, Monica – *Geraldine – for the Love of a Transvestite* (Caliban Books, 1988)

Rodway, Howard – *The Psychic Directory* (Futura, 1984)

Rodway, Howard – *Tarot of The Old Path* (Urania, Switzerland, 1990)

Rodway, Howard – *Tarot of Northern Shadows* (AGM AGMuller, Switzerland, 1998)

Rodway, Howard – *The Rune Vision Cards* (Vega, 2002)

Sex Guide International (Italy) Website www.sexy-guide.com

E-mail info@sexy-guide.com

Snake, Doktor – *Doktor Snake's Voodoo Spellbook* (Eddison Sadd Editions, 2000)

Two Worlds, Two Worlds Publishing, London.

Valiente, Doreen – *An ABC of Witchcraft Past and Present* (Robert Hale, 1973)

Vicky, Lee – *Transgender A –Z* (WayOut Publishing. Published annually)

Yarbro, Chelsea Quinn – *Messages from Michael* (Playboy Press, USA, 1979)

Yarbro, Chelsea Quinn – *More Messages from Michael* (Berkley Books, USA, 1986)

Yarbro, Chelsea Quinn – *Michael's People* (Berkley Books, USA, 1988)

At this time of writing some of the books, such as the *Michael* books, are out of print. Online second-hand book dealers such as *abebooks* may well have the volumes that you wish to obtain. Try at www.abebooks.com

Index

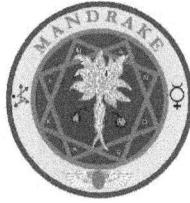

If you enjoyed this book
and want to know more
sign up for free Mandrake monthly book newsletter, here's how:
Visit the
mandrake.uk.net
website
A subscription page should pop-up

or type this link into a browser

http://eepurl.com/THE9P